AF540455

Animal Behaviour

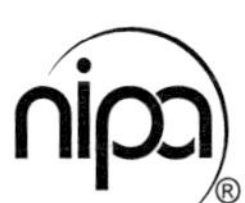

NIPA® GENX ELECTRONIC RESOURCES & SOLUTIONS P. LTD.
New Delhi-110 034

About the Editor

Dr. Tanmoy Rana obtained his Bachelor of Veterinary Sciences and Animal Husbandry degree (B.V.Sc. & A.H.) and Masters (M.V.Sc) in Veterinary Medicine, Ethics & Jurisprudence from West Bengal University of Animal and Fishery Sciences, Kolkata, India. He secured his Doctor of Philosophy (Ph.D.) in Veterinary Science from the University of Calcutta, Kolkata, India. He works currently as an Assistant Professor of the Veterinary Clinical Complex at West Bengal University of Animal and Fishery Sciences, Kolkata, India. Previously he has also worked as a Veterinary Officer, Animal Resources Development Department, Government of West Bengal, India. He is actively engaged in teaching and clinical practices in veterinary medicine and research related to animal health, production, and disease monitoring regimes. His research interests involve arsenic toxicity, molecular diagnosis, molecular toxicology and medicine, oxidative stress, immunopathology, nanoparticles, Echinococcosis, and microbes. He has published several research articles in reputed international and national journals along with review articles in international journals. He is an editorial board member (especially BMC Veterinary Research, Associate Editor of Frontier in Veterinary Science), and a reviewer of international and national journals. He is a member of many international scientific societies and organizations importantly the West Bengal Veterinary Council (WBVC), The Indian Society for Veterinary Medicine (ISVM), the Association of Public Health Veterinarians, and The Indian Science Congress Association (ISCA). He is also an associate of the West Bengal Academy of Science & Technology, West Bengal, India. He is an editor and author of so many national and international books.

Animal Behaviour

Tanmoy Rana Ph.D.AFWAST, FVASc.
Assistant Professor
Veterinary Clinical Complex
(Veterinary Medicine, Ethics & Jurisprudence)
Department of Veterinary Clinical Complex
West Bengal University of Animal & Fishery Sciences
Kolkata-700037, West Bengal, India

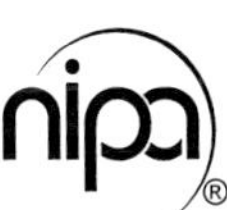

NIPA® GENX ELECTRONIC RESOURCES & SOLUTIONS P. LTD.
New Delhi-110 034

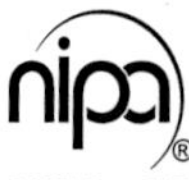

**NIPA® GENX ELECTRONIC
RESOURCES & SOLUTIONS P. LTD.**

101,103, Vikas Surya Plaza, CU Block
L.S.C. Market, Pitam Pura, New Delhi-110 034
Ph : +91-11-43860225, Mob.: +91 9717133558, 9540816132
E-mail: newindiapublishingagency@gmail.com
Website: www.nipaersources.com

Print ISBN: 978-93-58874-98-3

ebook ISBN: 978-93-58876-46-8

Composed and Designed by NIPA®.

Preface

This Key notes of Animal Behavior book presents all basic aspect of MCQ on animal behaviour in a very clear and concise format with updates. The book is designed to boost up students and job aspirants for the preparation of different examination like ICAR-JRF, SRF, NET, ARS, CSIR/ICMR-JRF, UPSC, State PSCs, PG and PhD Entrance and other competitive exams. The animal behavior book is fast becoming core and most important topic in the curriculum of agriculture and veterinary students. The MCQ book provides a rich resource for students as well as teachers from a wide range of life science disciplines. The MCQ is presented in a simple and lucid style for the easy understanding about the subject. Each chapter is well-supported by different contributors in their own expertise and serve the chapter in more interesting way.

The MCQ include its clear explanations and concise, readable text and the enthusiasm of the authors for their subject. All chapters of this book are scrupulously and nicely edited to keep it more interesting and easy retention of updated information in which reader can acquire recent knowledge about the subject. This book will be immense useful and aids an important resource to all students of veterinary college, academicians, paper setter, and job aspirants.

I hope the book helps the reader immensely.

Editor

Acknowledgement

I convey my sincere gratitude to Hon'ble Vice Chancellor, West Bengal University of Animal & Fishery Sciences for providing opportunity to edit the book. I am also helpful to all contributors who wholeheartedly helped me by sending their chapters in proper time. The special thanks goes to all colleagues for their useful ideas, and suggestion in this regard. I also convey sincere thanks to all the personnel at publisher for helping me with the opportunity to act as editor for this MCQ book. I am also grateful to family members for providing a great support and the time to finalize the book.

Editor

Contents

1

Introduction

Aravindh S.[1], Mohamed Hasif G.[2], Monalisha Debbarma[2] and Tanmoy Rana[3]

[1]*Department of Physiology, College of Veterinary and Animal Sciences Odisha University of Agriculture and Technology, Bhubaneshwar, Odisha*

[2]*Institute of Veterinary Science and Animal Husbandry, Siksha O Anusandhan University, Odisha*

[3]*Department of Veterinary Clinical Complex, West Bengal University of Animal & Fishery Sciences, Kolkata, West Bengal*

Introduction to Animal behavior

The tale of modern humans is a captivating narrative that begins around 200,000 years ago, marked by the practices of gathering and hunting wild animals. The advent of domestication heralded a new era, paving the way for diverse human societies, cultures, and traditions in what is known as the Neolithic transition. Domestication, an evolutionary process driven by genetic changes through artificial selection for human-beneficial traits and natural selection in captivity over numerous generations, reshaped the relationship between humans and animals. This intricate dance of evolution, genetics, and human ingenuity gave rise to an array of species adapted to human care and companionship. Fitness, in this context, refers to an animal's ability to thrive in close quarters with humans, conspecifics, and other animals, consume readily available food, breed successfully in captivity, and elicit human care in an anthropogenic setting. This adaptation process led to phenotypes characterized by reduced "fight or flight" responses, increased social tolerance, and less selectivity, enabling efficient use of available resources. Traits such as early sexual maturity, less seasonality in breeding, and, occasionally, pedomorphism—the retention of juvenile, playful behavior into adulthood—further illustrate the transformative effects of domestication.For terrestrial animals, three primary domestication routes have been identified: the commensal pathway, the prey pathway, and the direct route. In the commensal pathway, animals played a significant role in their domestication. Attracted by human waste, they initially settled in artificial environments, eventually forming mutually beneficial relationships with humans. Species such as the chicken (Gallus domesticus), cat (Felis catus), and dog (Canis familiaris) followed this pathway.

The prey pathway began with humans seeking to enhance the yield or predictability of resources like meat or hides, possibly due to the depletion of local prey stocks after extensive hunting. These management techniques gradually led to regulated breeding and, in some cases, the development of true herd management. Goats (Capra hircus), sheep

(Ovis aries), and cattle (Bos taurus) are prime examples of species domesticated through this pathway.The direct route involved humans intentionally setting out to tame specific species. This approach, starting with the deliberate capture of wild animals and aiming to control their reproduction, bypassed the early stages of habituation and management. Consequently, this pathway proceeded more rapidly and featured a significant bottleneck. Notable species domesticated via the direct route include the donkey (Equus asinus), the dromedary (Camelus dromedarius), and the horse (Equus caballus).

Historically, sheep were initially raised for their meat supply before human-mediated specialization for milk and wool began around 4,000–5,000 years ago. Goats, adaptable to arid, alpine, and tropical regions where other livestock would struggle, were domesticated around 10,000 years ago in the Fertile Crescent. The domestication of zebu cattle in the Indus Valley region occurred around 8,000–7,500 B.P., while taurine cattle were domesticated between 10,500 and 10,000 B.P. The now-extinct Equus ferus from central Asia is the wild ancestor of the domestic horse, with significant contributions to the genetic makeup of domestic horses from the Asian wild horse, Equus przewalskii.The study of animal behavior, an intriguing field, delves into the interactions and adaptations of animals. It correlates internal and external stimuli with the rate of change in their adaptations and actions. Feeding, grazing, and sexual behavior of different species play a crucial role in determining animal husbandry traits. Over the years, complex pathways of behavior activation have been explored. For instance, the plausible mechanism of oxytocin-induced release of dopamine by olfactory cells could aid a dam in recognizing her neonates.Compared to wolves, dogs exhibit a greater inclination to approach humans, have longer socialization periods, are more socially accepting, and can reproduce year-round, unlike the seasonal breeding of wolves. These behavioral differences are accompanied by morphological changes, such as smaller canines, less sexual dimorphism in canine length, and greater variation in body size, coat, ear, and tail form. Adult dogs also display pedomorphism, remaining lively and vocal like juveniles.Learning, a continuous process influenced by past and present experiences, significantly shapes animal behavior. It encompasses various types, including classical learning, operant learning, aversion, and maze learning. In captivity, learning plays a pivotal role in shaping a domestic phenotype, alongside genetic and epigenetic factors.

The fundamental research on behavioral, emotional, and cognitive reactions to domestication offers rich opportunities to understand the interplay between developmental and evolutionary processes. Understanding how animals adapt to different confinement settings has implications for both human and animal welfare. These include the efficiency of livestock production, the quality of biomedical data from animal models, and the success of companion animal adoption from shelters.Modeling connections between genotypic and phenotypic time-series data can advance our understanding of the evolutionary processes involved in domestication and feralization. Comparing phenotypic variance at different ages and habitats can provide insights into how experience and development contribute to domesticated traits. This comprehensive understanding can lead to improvements in animal husbandry, conservation efforts, and the overall welfare of both domesticated and wild species.

MCQ's

1. How do cows cope with heat stress during the summer season?
   a) Decrease water intake b) Increase respiration rate
   c) Seek direct sunlight d) Avoid shaded areas
2. What is the role of oxytocin in milk production in animals?
   a) Inhibits milk letdown
   b) Stimulates adrenaline release
   c) Increases milk production
   d) Causes discomfort
3. How do horses regulate their body temperature during hot weather?
   a) Decrease water intake b) Graze during midday heat
   c) Rest during cooler temperatures d) Sweat extensively
4. How do birds regulate their body temperature during hot weather?
   a) Fluffing up their feathers b) Panting
   c) Huddling together d) Sunbathing
5. Why is access to fresh, clean water crucial for birds during hot weather?
   a) To build nests b) To attract mates
   c) To regulate their body temperature d) To find food
6. What is the purpose of birds increasing their breathing rate during hot weather?
   a) To conserve energy
   b) To scare off predators
   c) To evaporate water from their respiratory system
   d) To communicate with other birds
7. What is the term used for the process of giving birth in dogs and wolves?
   a) Farrowing b) Calving
   c) Whelping d) Kindling
8. What is the term for the process of giving birth in lions, tigers, and leopards?
   a) Farrowing b) Calving
   c) Whelping d) Cubbing
9. What is the purpose of nursing in mammalian mothers?
   a) To provide shelter for the newborns
   b) To teach the newborns survival skills
   c) To feed the newborns with milk produced by mammary glands
   d) To discipline the newborns
10. What distinguishes seasonal breeders from continuous breeders?
    a) Seasonal breeders reproduce throughout the year
    b) Continuous breeders reproduce only at a specific time of year
    c) Seasonal breeders reproduce at a particular period in a year
    d) Continuous breeders reproduce sporadically

11. Which type of breeding pattern do animals fall into if they reproduce at various times throughout the year?
    a) Seasonal breeders
    b) Continuous breeders
    c) Sporadic breeders
    d) Periodic breeders
12. What characterizes continuous breeders in terms of their reproductive behavior?
    a) They reproduce only once in their lifetime
    b) They reproduce at a specific time every year
    c) They reproduce in response to environmental cues
    d) They reproduce at random intervals
13. What is the primary reason for ovulation in female animals?
    a) Increased aggression
    b) Environmental factors
    c) Dominance
    d) Hormones
14. How do male elephants behave during musth?
    a) They engage in combat dances
    b) They curl back their lips to sense pheromones
    c) They mate with multiple females
    d) They sniff the cow's urine
15. What is the purpose of the flehmen response in horses?
    a) To engage in combat dances
    b) To sense pheromones in the environment
    c) To wrestle for dominance
    d) To pass on genes
16. What stimulates the process of spermatogenesis in males at puberty?
    a) Release of estrogen
    b) Release of progesterone
    c) Release of testosterone
    d) Release of oxytocin
17. Which animal species reaches puberty the earliest based on the provided data?
    a) Horse
    b) Cattle
    c) Pig
    d) Cat
18. What is the main purpose of the Flehmen Response displayed by bulls?
    a) To intimidate other males
    b) To communicate with other bulls
    c) To attract females for mating
    d) To mark territory
19. Which animals are primarily grazers?
    a) Dogs and cats
    b) Horses and zebras
    c) Birds and reptiles
    d) Fish and amphibians
20. How do animals cope with seasonal changes?
    a) By swimming in water bodies
    b) By migrating to warmer regions
    c) By seeking shade in summer and huddling for warmth in winter
    d) By hibernating throughout the year

21. What is the function of the rumen in ruminant ungulates?
    a) Absorption of nutrients
    b) Storage of food
    c) Initial digestion of food
    d) Regulation of body temperature
22. Which chamber of the ruminant ungulate's stomach is responsible for absorbing water and electrolytes?
    a) Rumen
    b) Reticulum
    c) Omasum
    d) Abomasum
23. How do ruminant ungulates efficiently digest fibrous plant materials?
    a) By secreting enzymes in the stomach
    b) By regurgitating and re-chewing food
    c) By having a single-chambered stomach
    d) By consuming only animal-based foods
24. What is the primary focus of the field of "Physiology of Behaviour"?
    a) Understanding how plants grow
    b) Exploring the relationship between brain function and behavior
    c) Studying the history of animal husbandry
    d) Investigating the effects of climate change on ecosystems
25. Why are feeding, grazing, and sexual behaviors extensively studied in animal husbandry?
    a) Due to their impact on mental health disorders
    b) Because they are unrelated to the economics of animal husbandry
    c) Direct correlation with the economics of animal husbandry
    d) To understand the impact of climate change on animal behavior
26. What distinguishes ruminant ungulates from non-ruminants in terms of feeding behavior?
    a) They have a single-chambered stomach
    b) They possess a multi-chambered stomach
    c) They primarily feed on insects
    d) They have a specialized digestive system for meat
27. What behavior is commonly observed in pregnant cows close to calving?
    a) Increased activity levels
    b) Decreased appetite
    c) Nesting behaviors
    d) Aggressive behavior towards other cows
28. How do mares typically behave as gestation progresses?
    a) Increased willingness to engage in strenuous exercise
    b) Decreased levels of activity
    c) Reduced protective instincts
    d) Decreased food intake

29. What is a common behavior observed in pregnant elephants near the end of the gestation period?
    a) Increased aggression towards other elephants
    b) Decreased food consumption
    c) Displaying more maternal behaviors
    d) Seeking isolation from the herd
30. What are some signs that a pregnant dog (bitch) is preparing to give birth?
    a) Increased appetite and hyperactivity
    b) Enlarged abdomen and mammary glands
    c) Loss of fur and decreased water intake
    d) Aggressive behavior and excessive barking
31. Why do pregnant dogs (bitches) start nesting before giving birth?
    a) To find a mate for their puppies
    b) To prepare a safe and comfortable space for birthing
    c) To escape from potential predators
    d) To search for food for their newborns
32. What is a common behavior observed in pregnant dogs (bitches) as they approach labor?
    a) Increased socialization with other animals
    b) Decreased need for rest and sleep
    c) Seeking a quiet and secure place to give birth
    d) Aggressive behavior towards their owners
33. What distinguishes seasonal breeders from continuous breeders?
    a) Seasonal breeders can mate throughout the year, while continuous breeders breed at a particular period.
    b) Seasonal breeders include humans, rats, and cats, while continuous breeders include deer, birds, and sheep.
    c) Seasonal breeders exhibit signs of standing heat, while continuous breeders show frequent urination.
    d) Seasonal breeders are aggressive towards males, while continuous breeders show nesting behavior.
34. Which animal behavior is NOT typically associated with the gestation period?
    a) Building the maternal nest
    b) Increased vocalization
    c) More intake of feed
    d) Restlessness during or before parturition
35. What is a common behavior exhibited by dogs during heat?
    a) Increased affection towards males
    b) Frequent rolling
    c) Signs of swollen vulva
    d) Nesting behavior

36. What dental adaptations do grazers typically have for their feeding behavior?
    a) Sharp canines for gripping prey
    b) Narrow teeth for cutting leaves and twigs
    c) Pronounced incisors for nipping meat
    d) Wide, flat teeth for grinding tough grasses

37. Which animal is known for its browsing behavior, feeding on leaves, branches, and shrubs?
    a) Horses b) Zebras
    c) White rhinoceroses d) Black rhinoceroses

38. What type of stomach do horses have that aids in breaking down fibrous materials during grazing?
    a) Multi-chambered stomach b) Simple stomach
    c) Hindgut fermentation d) Rumen fermentation

39. What is a common feeding behavior seen in carnivorous animals due to their evolutionary adaptations?
    a) Grazing on grasses b) Browsing on leaves and shrubs
    c) Hunting and consuming prey d) Rotting in swine

40. What is a key characteristic of ruminant ungulates that aids in the digestion of fibrous plant materials?
    a) Single-chambered stomach b) Hindgut fermentation
    c) Multi-chambered stomach d) Salivary digestion

41. Which of the following animals is known for primarily browsing on leaves, twigs, and fruits from shrubs and trees?
    a) Cattle b) Sheep
    c) Deer d) Giraffes

42. What distinguishes non-ruminant ungulates from ruminant ungulates in terms of their digestive system?
    a) They have a multi-chambered stomach
    b) They rely on hindgut fermentation
    c) They chew cud
    d) They have a simple stomach structure

43. Which animal is an example of browsing behavior, feeding on a variety of plant materials including grasses, shrubs, and tree leaves?
    a) Cattle b) Sheep
    c) Deer d) Goats

44. What physical adaptation allows giraffes to feed on leaves, flowers, and fruits from tall trees?
    a) Wide mouths b) Strong tongues
    c) Long necks d) Multi-chambered stomach

45. How do birds maintain body heat in cold temperatures?
   a) Fluffing up their feathers
   b) Drinking cold water
   c) Flying higher in the sky
   d) Eating more food
46. What is a common strategy for elephants to keep warm in cold weather?
   a) Swimming in cold water
   b) Rolling in the snow
   c) Increasing their activity levels
   d) Hiding in caves
47. What are some emotional indicators in animals?
   a) Swimming patterns
   b) Vocalizations like barking
   c) Climbing trees
   d) Hibernating in winter
48. What are some of the emotions that primates, including humans, are known to display
   a) Excitement
   b) Surprise
   c) Disgust
   d) Sadness
49. How do primates often establish social bonds?
   a) Through vocalizations
   b) Through aggressive behaviors
   c) Through grooming and other affiliative behaviors
   d) Through territorial displays
50. Which primate species is known for expressing emotions like joy, sadness, anger, and fear?
   a) Orangutans
   b) Gorillas
   c) Baboons
   d) Chimpanzees
51. How do birds regulate their body temperature during hot weather?
   a) Fluffing their feathers
   b) Panting
   c) Huddling together
   d) Basking in the sun
52. What is a common thermoregulation method used by elephants during summer?
   a) Flapping their ears
   b) Rolling in mud
   c) Panting
   d) Huddling together
53. How do horses maintain body heat during winter?
   a) Panting
   b) Growing a thick winter coat
   c) Bathing in water
   d) Consuming less forage
54. How do dogs typically express happiness?
   a) Purring and kneading
   b) Hiding and cowering
   c) Jumping, wagging their tails, and barking excitedly
   d) Continuously barking or biting

55. What emotional behavior is commonly seen in parrots when separated from their mates or flock?
    a) Purring
    b) Hissing
    c) Displaying vocal and physical signs of distress
    d) Continuously barking

56. How do cats typically show contentment?
    a) Hugging
    b) Purring and kneading
    c) Cowering
    d) Continuously barking

57. What is a key feature of software designed for assessing behavioral studies?
    a) Emphasis on rigidity and fixed structures
    b) Focus on simplicity and limited functionality
    c) Prioritization of flexibility, scalability, and accuracy
    d) Dependence on manual data entry

58. What role do algorithms play in modern human-computer interactions?
    a) Algorithms are obsolete and not used in modern interactions
    b) Algorithms are used sparingly due to their inefficiency
    c) Algorithms are crucial in assisting and enhancing human-computer interactions
    d) Algorithms hinder the effectiveness of human-computer interactions

59. What is a significant factor that influences the success of dogs utilizing their olfactory cells?
    a) Temperature
    b) Humidity
    c) Sex
    d) Age

60. What is the proven effect of oxytocin on various social behaviors in animals?
    a) Milk secretion
    b) Reproductive function
    c) Formation of social bonds
    d) Digestive system regulation

61. What is a pivotal advance in the field of animal behavior related to earthquake prediction?
    a) Detection of seismo-electromagnetic precursors
    b) Changes in bird migration patterns
    c) Increase in fish population
    d) Growth of plant species

62. What gene was identified as a potential candidate for tame behavior in foxes in the genome-wide analysis?
    a) FoxR1
    b) SorCS1
    c) Vulpes1
    d) AMPA1

63. What specific area of study is being potentially impacted by animal behavior research?
    a) Space exploration
    b) Earthquake prediction
    c) Botany
    d) Historical events analysis

64. How do honeybees communicate with their members?
    a) By singing
    b) By performing specific dance sequences
    c) By emitting pheromones
    d) By using visual signals
65. How does exogenous oxytocin affect dogs?
    a) It enhances their sense of taste
    b) It increases their gaze towards humans
    c) It improves their hearing abilities
    d) It boosts their sense of touch
66. What potential benefits can be derived from studying the behavioral, emotional, and cognitive reactions to domestication?
    a) Improved understanding of animal communication
    b) Enhanced comprehension of developmental and evolutionary processes
    c) Increased agricultural productivity
    d) Better weather prediction models
67. How can modeling connections between genotypic and phenotypic time-series data contribute to understanding domestication and feralization?
    a) Predicting future climate change patterns
    b) Identifying new species of animals
    c) Advancing knowledge of evolutionary processes
    d) Improving smartphone technology
68. How can comparing phenotypic variance at different ages and habitats aid in comprehending domesticated traits?
    a) Enhancing space exploration technology
    b) Improving agricultural irrigation systems
    c) Understanding the role of experience and development in trait development
    d) Developing new energy sources
69. What role does the interplay between developmental and evolutionary processes play in the success rate of companion animal adoption from shelters?
    a) Influencing the growth of social media platforms
    b) Affecting the behavior and adaptability of animals in new environments
    c) Determining the price of pet supplies
    d) Shaping global economic policies
70. How can advancements in understanding domestication benefit both cattle production and biomedical research?
    a) Enhancing the quality of online shopping experiences
    b) Improving the efficiency of transportation systems
    c) Increasing the effectiveness of cattle production and biomedical data derived from nn animal models
    d) Boosting the tourism industry

71. What factors contributed to the successful adaptation of goats to arid, alpine, and tropical regions?
    a) Their ability to thrive in cold climates
    b) Their preference for dense forests
    c) Their resistance to extreme temperatures and limited food sources
    d) Their need for constant access to water
72. How did the domestication of zebu cattle impact the Indus valley region around 8000–7500 B.P.?
    a) It led to a decrease in agricultural productivity
    b) It facilitated the development of trade routes
    c) It caused a decline in the population of other livestock species
    d) It resulted in the establishment of permanent settlements
73. Which wild ancestor is the domestic horse descended from?
    a) Equus przewalskii
    b) Equus ferus
    c) Equus caballus
    d) Equus zebra
74. What role did the Asian wild horse, Equus przewalskii, play in the genetic composition of domestic horses?
    a) It contributed significantly to their genetic diversity
    b) It caused a decrease in their overall population
    c) It led to the extinction of certain horse breeds
    d) It had no impact on the genetic makeup of domestic horses
75. How did the domestication of taurine cattle around 10,500–10,000 B.P. impact human societies?
    a) It led to a decrease in agricultural practices
    b) It facilitated the development of advanced irrigation systems
    c) It caused a shift towards a nomadic lifestyle
    d) It resulted in the establishment of permanent settlements
76. In what ways did the domestication of sheep differ from that of goats?
    a) Sheep were primarily raised for their milk supply
    b) Sheep were domesticated in tropical regions
    c) Sheep were adapted to arid climates
    d) Sheep were initially raised for their meat supply
77. How did the domestication of livestock species impact the development of early human civilizations?
    a) It led to a decrease in human population growth
    b) It facilitated the establishment of trade networks
    c) It caused a decline in agricultural productivity
    d) It resulted in the abandonment of settled communities

78. What role does oxytocin play in the recognition of neonates by a dam?
    a) Stimulating feeding behavior
    b) Inducing release of dopamine by olfactory cells
    c) Regulating mating behavior
    d) Controlling territorial aggression
79. How do dogs differ from wolves in terms of social behavior?
    a) Wolves are more gregarious than dogs
    b) Dogs have a shorter socialization window than wolves
    c) Dogs are less tolerant of social interactions compared to wolves
    d) Dogs can reproduce year-round while wolves show seasonality
80. What is a key difference in the morphological characteristics between dogs and wolves?
    a) Wolves have smaller canines than dogs
    b) Dogs show more sexual dimorphism in body size
    c) Wolves have greater variance in coat, ear, and tail form
    d) Dogs display less sexual dimorphism in canine length
81. How does learning contribute to shaping a domestic phenotype in animals?
    a) By altering genetic makeup
    b) By influencing social behavior
    c) By modifying physical appearance
    d) By combining with genetic and epigenetic factors
82. In what ways does operant learning differ from classical learning?
    a) Operant learning involves involuntary responses, while classical learning involves voluntary actions
    b) Operant learning focuses on rewards and punishments, while classical learning is based on associations
    c) Operant learning is based on instinct, while classical learning is based on conditioning
    d) Operant learning is used for social behaviors, while classical learning is used for survival instincts
83. How does the socialization window of dogs impact their behavior compared to wolves?
    a) Dogs are less tolerant of social interactions due to a shorter window
    b) Wolves have a longer socialization window leading to more gregarious behavior
    c) Dogs are more accepting of social interactions due to a longer window
    d) Wolves show more aggression in social situations because of a shorter window

84. What is the significance of the activation of a behavior pathway in animals?
   a) It determines their mating preferences
   b) It influences their feeding habits
   c) It regulates their social interactions
   d) It correlates with their adaptations and actions

85. What potential ethical considerations should be taken into account when discussing the deliberate capture of wild animals to reduce their reproduction?
   a) Increased risk of disease transmission
   b) Impact on genetic diversity
   c) Potential disruption of ecosystems
   d) Decreased competition for resources

86. How might the deliberate capture of wild animals for population control impact the overall biodiversity of an ecosystem?
   a) Increase in species richness
   b) Decrease in habitat fragmentation
   c) Disruption of predator-prey relationships
   d) Promotion of genetic variation

87. In what ways could the deliberate capture of wild animals for population control lead to unintended consequences in the ecosystem?
   a) Enhanced species resilience
   b) Accelerated adaptation to environmental changes
   c) Disruption of natural selection processes
   d) Promotion of species coexistence

88. What distinguishes the commensal pathway of animal domestication from the prey pathway and the directed route?
   a) Animals are intentionally captured for breeding
   b) Animals are attracted by human waste and form mutually beneficial relationships
   c) Animals are primarily used for meat or hides
   d) Animals are managed in regulated herds

89. How did the prey pathway of animal domestication differ from the commensal approach?
   a) Animals were attracted by human settlements
   b) Animals were intentionally captured for breeding purposes
   c) Animals formed mutually beneficial relationships with humans
   d) Animals were primarily used for labor

90. Which animals primarily followed the directed route of domestication?
   a) Cats, dogs, and chickens
   b) Goats, sheep, and cattle
   c) Donkeys, dromedaries, & horses
   d) Elephants, zebras, & giraffes

91. In the context of animal domestication, what is the significance of the bottleneck effect in the direct route?
    a) It led to the depletion of local prey animal stocks
    b) It accelerated the process of taming wild animals
    c) It resulted in the creation of true herd management
    d) It attracted animals to human settlements

92. How did the commensal pathway of animal domestication involve a symbiotic relationship between animals and humans?
    a) Animals were primarily used for labor
    b) Animals were attracted by human waste and formed mutually beneficial relationships
    c) Animals were intentionally captured for breeding purposes
    d) Animals were managed in regulated herds

93. What role did human waste play in the commensal pathway of animal domestication?
    a) It attracted animals to human settlements
    b) It served as a source of food for domesticated animals
    c) It accelerated the taming process of wild animals
    d) It led to the depletion of local prey animal stocks

94. How did the prey pathway of animal domestication contribute to the development of regulated breeding and herd management?
    a) By attracting animals to human settlements
    b) By forming mutually beneficial relationships with animals
    c) By intentionally capturing animals for breeding purposes
    d) By depleting local prey animal stocks

95. In what ways does the concept of fitness play a role in the domestication process?
    a) Fitness refers to the ability to avoid human care in an anthropogenic setting
    b) Fitness involves the ability to consume scarce food resources
    c) Fitness includes the ability to survive in close quarters with people and other animals, consume readily available food, and successfully breed in captivity
    d) Fitness is unrelated to the domestication process

96. How do traits like decreased "fight or flight" reactions and increased social tolerance contribute to the domestication process?
    a) They hinder the ability of animals to adapt to captivity
    b) They promote aggression towards humans
    c) They enable effective use of available resources and interaction with humans
    d) They have no impact on the domestication process

97. What role does pedomorphism play in the domestication process?
    a) It leads to increased aggression in domesticated animals
    b) It results in delayed sexual maturity
    c) It involves the continuation of youthful, playful behavior into adulthood
    d) It has no impact on the domestication process

98. How does the Neolithic transition relate to the concept of domestication?
    a) The Neolithic transition led to a decrease in domesticated animal populations
    b) The Neolithic transition marked the development of various human societies, cultures, and traditions through domestication
    c) The Neolithic transition had no impact on the domestication process
    d) The Neolithic transition focused solely on hunting wild animals

99. What are some potential implications of the domestication process on human-animal interactions in modern society?
    a) Increased aggression in domesticated animals towards humans
    b) Enhanced social tolerance in domesticated animals leading to better human-animal relationships
    c) Decreased availability of resources for domesticated animals
    d) No impact on human-animal interactions

100. Which of the following neurotransmitters is primarily responsible for cessation of food intake in animals?
    a) Dopamine
    b) Serotonin
    c) Cholecystokinin (CCK)
    d) Ghrelin

101. Which osmoreceptors, when activated, lead to a decrease in food intake in animals?
    a) Area postrema osmoreceptors
    b) Anteroventral third ventricle (AV3V) region osmoreceptors
    c) Subfornical organ (SFO) osmoreceptors
    d) Carotid sinus osmoreceptors

102. What hormone is produced by adipose tissue (fat cells) that regulates energy balance and body weight?
    a) Insulin
    b) Leptin
    c) Ghrelin
    d) Melatonin

103. Which of the following genes interact with LEPR to regulate energy balance, food intake, and body weight?
    a) LEP, MC4R, POMC, NPY, AgRP
    b) LEP, MC4R, POMC only
    c) NPY, AgRP only
    d) None of the above

104. What is the function of the LEPR gene?
    a) To produce leptin
    b) To regulate food intake and metabolism
    c) To provide instructions for making the leptin receptor
    d) To transmit signals to the brain

105. Which of the following mechanisms plays a crucial role in animal's ability to detect and respond to nutrient deficiencies or excesses in their diet?
   a) Gut-brain axis signaling
   b) Hormonal regulation (e.g. insulin, leptin)
   c) Nutrient-sensing pathways (e.g. mTOR, AMPK)
   d) All of the above

106. What is the most potent external factor that influences feeding behavior in animals?
   a) Food availability
   b) Food palatability
   c) Social influences
   d) Environmental temperature

107. Which of the following is a possible reason for intestinal stretching in horses?
   a) Overeating
   b) Under-eating
   c) Gastrointestinal disorder
   d) Behavioral adaptation

108. What is the primary role of cyproheptadine in animals?
   a) To decrease feed intake
   b) To stimulate appetite and increase feed intake
   c) To improve feed efficiency
   d) To reduce stress

109. Which hormone is involved in social bonding and attachment, contributing to proceptive behavior?
   a) Oxytocin
   b) Dopamine
   c) Estrogen
   d) Progesterone

110. Which hormone is responsible for helping a ewe recognize her lamb?
   a) Oxytocin
   b) Prolactin
   c) Vasopressin
   d) Estrogen

111. What term describes the maternal behaviour in animals where a mother curves her body around her offspring to provide protection, warmth, and comfort?
   a) Convexation
   b) Concaveation
   c) Curvation
   d) Incurvation

112. Which type of reinforcement involves adding a pleasing stimulus after desired behavior?
   a) Positive Reinforcement
   b) Negative Reinforcement
   c) Primary Reinforcement
   d) Secondary Reinforcement

113. Which site is most closely associated with spatial memory in animals?
   a) Hippocampus
   b) Amygdala
   c) Cerebellum
   d) Prefrontal cortex

114. Which site plays a role in motor learning in animals?
   a) Cerebellum
   b) Hippocampus
   c) Amygdala
   d) Prefrontal cortex

115. Which receptor is primarily involved in associative memory in dogs?
    a) NMDA b) AMPAR
    c) Acetylcholine d) Dopamine

116. Which receptor is involved in spatial memory and is also responsible for the formation and consolidation of new memories in dogs?
    a) NMDA b) AMPAR
    c) Dopamine d) Acetylcholine

117. What is the impact of 5HT1A gene polymorphisms on serotonin signaling in dogs?
    a) Increased serotonin signaling
    b) Decreased serotonin signaling
    c) No effect on serotonin signaling
    d) Variable effect on serotonin signaling

118. What is the association between polymorphisms in the 5HT1A gene and behavior in dogs?
    a) Polymorphisms are associated with increased aggression
    b) Polymorphisms are associated with decreased anxiety
    c) Polymorphisms are associated with increased fear-based behaviors
    d) Polymorphisms are associated with decreased social behavior

Answer Key

1	b	2	c	3	d	4	b	5	c	6	c	7	c
8	d	9	c	10	c	11	b	12	c	13	d	14	c
15	b	16	c	17	c	18	c	19	b	20	c	21	c
22	c	23	b	24	b	25	c	26	b	27	c	28	b
29	c	30	b	31	b	32	c	33	a	34	b	35	c
36	d	37	d	38	b	39	c	40	c	41	c	42	b
43	d	44	c	45	a	46	c	47	b	48	d	49	c
50	d	51	b	52	a	53	b	54	c	55	c	56	b
57	c	58	c	59	d	60	c	61	a	62	b	63	b
64	b	65	b	66	b	67	c	68	c	69	b	70	c
71	c	72	b	73	b	74	a	75	d	76	d	77	b
78	b	79	d	80	d	81	d	82	b	83	c	84	d
85	b	86	c	87	c	88	b	89	b	90	c	91	b
92	b	93	a	94	d	95	c	96	c	97	c	98	b
99	b	100	c	101	c	102	b	103	a	104	c	105	d
106	a	107	d	108	b	109	a	110	a	111	b	112	a
113	a	114	a	115	c	116	a	117	b	118	c		

2

Animal Behaviour During Restraining Handling and Feeding

Shashi Pradhan[1], Ranbir Singh Jatav[1], Riya Mathur[2] and Harsit Kaur Sachdeva[2]

College of Veterinary Sciences and Animal Husbandry, Nanaji Deshmukh Veterinary Sciences University, Jabalpur, Madhya Pardesh

Introduction

The behaviour of animals during restraining, handling, and feeding is a crucial aspect of animal husbandry and veterinary care. Understanding and interpreting their behaviour in these contexts is essential for ensuring the well-being of animals and the safety of humans involved in their care.

I. Animal Behaviour During Restraining

1. **Fear and Anxiety:** When animals are restrained, they often exhibit fear and anxiety. This behaviour can manifest as vocalizations, attempts to escape, increased heart rate, and sometimes aggressive actions. Understanding the signs of fear and anxiety in animals is essential to mitigate stress during restraint. Calm and gentle handling can help reduce the negative impact on the animal's well-being.
2. **Fight or Flight Response Animals:** When restrained, may respond with a "fight or flight" reaction. They may try to flee or become defensive, potentially causing harm to themselves or the handlers. It is essential to anticipate this response and use appropriate restraints, such as halters or cages, to ensure safety for both animals and handlers.

II. Animal Behaviour During Handling

1. **Trust and Bonding:** The behaviour of animals during handling can vary depending on their previous experiences and the quality of their relationship with their caregivers. Animals that trust their handlers and have positive associations with handling are more likely to exhibit calm and cooperative behaviour. Trust is built through consistent, gentle, and respectful handling over time.
2. **Aggression and Fear:** Animals that have had negative handling experiences may exhibit aggression, avoidance, or fear during handling. This can pose risks to both the animals and the handlers. In such cases, it is essential to employ behaviour modification techniques and gradually desensitize the animals to handling procedures.

III. Animal Behaviour During Feeding

1. **Food Aggression:** Food is a potent motivator for most animals, and food aggression can be a significant behavioural issue during feeding. Dominant individuals may display aggressive behaviours to establish and defend their access to food. Careful feeding management, such as separate feeding areas or timed feedings, can mitigate these behaviours.
2. **Social Hierarchy:** In group-housed animals, feeding can reveal their social hierarchy. Dominant animals may feed first, and subordinate ones may wait their turn. Observing and understanding these behaviours can help ensure that all animals receive their fair share of food.
3. **Environmental Enrichment:** Feeding time can also serve as an opportunity for environmental enrichment. Providing food in puzzle feeders or through foraging activities can engage the animals' natural behaviours and stimulate their minds, promoting overall well-being.

Animal behaviour during restraining, handling, and feeding is a complex and dynamic field that requires careful observation and interpretation. Respectful and ethical practices are essential for promoting the well-being of animals and ensuring the safety of those involved in their care. By understanding and responding to the behavioural cues exhibited by animals, we can create a positive and secure environment for both animals and their caregivers, ultimately improving the quality of life for animals in our care. Animal behaviour is the study of how animals interact with their environment, with each other and how they respond to various stimuli. It encompasses a wide range of topics and can be studied in many different ways, from field observations to controlled experiments.

Here are some key aspects of animal behaviour

1. **Ethology**: Ethology is the scientific study of animal behavior, particularly in their natural environments. Ethologists observe and describe behaviors, seeking to understand their functions and evolution.
2. **Instinct and Learning**: Animals often exhibit a combination of instinctual (innate) behaviours and learned behaviours. Instinctual behaviours are genetically programmed, while learned behaviours are acquired through experience.
3. **Communication**: Animals communicate with each other through various means, including vocalizations, body language, pheromones, and visual displays. Communication serves purposes like mating, warning of danger, and social bonding.
4. **Social Behaviour**: Many species are social animals, living in groups or communities. Social behaviours include cooperation, competition, and various forms of hierarchy and dominance.
5. **Reproductive Behaviour**: Animals have evolved various strategies for reproduction, including courtship rituals, mating systems, and parenting behaviours.
6. **Foraging and Feeding**: How animals find, capture, and consume food is a critical aspect of their behaviour. This can involve solitary hunting, group hunting, or scavenging.
7. **Migration**: Some animals undertake long-distance migrations for purposes like breeding, feeding, or escaping unfavourable environmental conditions.

8. **Territorial Behavior**: Many animals establish and defend territories, which can be important for access to resources or mates.
9. **Learning and Cognition**: Some animals exhibit complex learning and problem-solving abilities. This includes tool use, spatial memory and the ability to adapt to new situations.
10. **Habituation and Sensitization**: Animals can become habituated to stimuli that are repeated and lose responsiveness, or they can become sensitized to stimuli and become more responsive over time.
11. **Aggression and Defence**: Animals may exhibit aggressive behaviours in various contexts, such as defending their territory, competing for mates or protecting their young.
12. **Sensory Perception**: Understanding how animals perceive the world through their senses (sight, hearing, smell, touch, and taste) is essential for comprehending their behaviour.
13. **Biological Rhythms**: Many animals have daily and seasonal rhythms that affect their behaviour, such as circadian rhythms and hibernation.
14. **Environmental Influences**: External factors like temperature, light and food availability can have a profound impact on animal behaviour.
15. **Human Impact**: Human activities, including habitat destruction, pollution, and climate change, can disrupt animal behaviour and ecosystems.

The study of animal behaviour is a multidisciplinary field that draws from biology, ecology, psychology, and ethology, among other disciplines. Researchers seek to understand the mechanisms and evolutionary reasons behind various behaviours and how they contribute to an animal's survival and reproduction. This knowledge has applications in wildlife conservation, animal welfare and even the understanding of human behaviour.

MCQ's

1. What are the objectives of Ethology?
   a) To achieve the animal welfare
   b) To know the main causes of abnormal behaviour
   c) Both
   d) None of the above
2. Grazing, feeding, drinking, rumination, suckling involves which type of pattern of behaviour?
   a) Eliminative   b) Ingestive
   c) Epimeletic behaviour   d) None
3. Which type of eating behaviour a horse shows?
   a) Bites or crops their food by upper & lower incisors
   b) Scoops by broad bills
   c) Wrapping a mouthful of grasses by their tongue
   d) None

4. Which type of eating behaviour a ruminant shows?
   a) Bites or crops their food by upper & lower incisors
   b) Scoops by broad bills
   c) Wrapping a mouthful of grasses by their tongue
   d) None

5. What is the feeding time of dog & cat?
   a) Both b) Once day in short time
   c) Large amount in short time d) None

6. What is the feeding time of ruminants?
   a) More time b) Short time
   c) Both d) None

7. In ingestive behaviour, it varies according to?
   a) Time of feeding
   b) Anatomy & physiology of animal
   c) Productivity & selectability
   d) All

8. Urination, defecation, body care involve which type of pattern of behaviour?
   a) Eliminative b) Ingestive
   c) Epimeletic d) None

9. Which animal is learns to bury faeces & urine?
   a) Cat b) Dog
   c) Both d) None

10. What is the meaning of Epimeletic behaviour?
    a) Aggression b) Care giving
    c) Both d) None

11. For puppies, Et- epimeletic behaviour is-
    a) Bleat b) Blow
    c) Whine d) None

12. For calves, Et- epimeletic behaviour is –
    a) Bleat b) Blow
    c) Whine d) None

13. What are the types of animal communications?
    a) Visual b) Auditory
    c) Tactile d) All

14. What are the behaviour disorder in horse?
    a) Kicking b) Biting
    c) Weaning d) All

15. What are the behaviour disorder in cattle?
    a) Tongue rolling b) Crib biting
    c) Both d) None

16. How much amount of water a buffalo require daily?
   a) 20 litres b) 40 litres
   c) 30 liters d) 25 liters
17. How much amount of water a sheep require daily in summer?
   a) 7-10 litres b) 10-15 litres
   c) Both d) None
18. What are the behaviour disorder in sheep?
   a) Wool pulling b) Wool eating
   c) Both d) None
19. By what transportation method a cattle is transported?
   a) By roadways b) By railway
   c) Both d) None
20. For short journey, how much days taken for transportation?
   a) up to 15 days b) up to days
   c) up to 20 days d) None
21. At what age, a young lambs begins wool eating (vices)?
   a) 2 or 4 weeks of age b) 1 or 2 weeks of age
   c) 3 or 4 weeks of age d) 4 or 5 weeks of age
22. Which animal is considered as sweeper animal (eat after harvesting)?
   a) Goat b) Sheep
   c) Both d) None
23. How much amount of water a cattle require daily?
   a) 14 litres b) 10 litres
   c) 20 litres d) None
24. What is the feeling time of camel?
   a) Large amount in a short time b) Small amount in a short time
   c) Both d) None
25. For calves, Et-epimeletic behaviour is-
   a) Bleat b) Blow
   c) Whine d) None
26. For lambs, Et-epimeletic behaviour is-
   a) Bleat b) Blow
   c) Whine d) None
27. What are the factors affecting the behaviour and management of animal?
   a) Species b) Breed
   c) Individuality d) All
28. What is the general temperament of dairy cattle?
   a) Nervous & excitable b) Dull & lymphatic
   c) Vicious & dangerous d) Docile or sweet

29. What is the general temperament of fattening animal?
   a) Nervous & excitable   b) Dull & lymphatic
   c) Vicious & dangerous   d) Docile or sweet
30. What is the general temperament of arabian horse?
   a) Nervous & excitable   b) Dull & lymphatic
   c) Vicious & dangerous   d) Docile or sweet
31. Which animal learns to urinate in special site (scent post)?
   a) Cat   b) Dog
   c) Both   d) None
32. Which animal does licking for body care?
   a) Cattle   b) Horse
   c) Cat   d) a & c
33. Which animal does rubbing for body care?
   a) Horse   b) Ruminant
   c) Cat   d) None
34. Which animal does scratching for body care?
   a) Horse   b) Ruminant
   c) Cat   d) None
35. What are the factors affecting ingestive behaviour of horse?
   a) Types of diet   b) Palatability
   c) Temperature   d) All
36. Which animal stops all body activities during defecation?
   a) Horse   b) Dog
   c) Both   d) None
37. How many times horse defecate per day?
   a) 12-20 times/day   b) 6-12 times/day
   c) 5-6 times/day   d) 20-24 times/day
38. Which animal shows tail lashes with left one leg (visual) characteristic ?
   a) Horse   b) Both
   c) Dog   d) None
39. What is the average time spent in grazing of cattle ?
   a) 2 to4 hr   b) 10 to 12 hr
   c) 4 to 9 hr   d) None
40. At what age calves begin to ruminate ?
   a) 2- 5 wk of age   b) 10 -12 wk of age
   c) 6-8 wk of age   d) None
41. What is the time of rumination per day approximately?
   a) 1/3 of grazing time   b) 3/4 of grazing time
   c) 1/4 of grazing time   d) None

42. How many time a cattle defeated per day?
    a) 10/ day b) 12 / day
    c) Both d) None
43. How many time a cattle urinate per day ?
    a) 9/ day b) 14/day
    c) 12 / day d) None
44. What Is the important of body of care?
    a) Decrease chance of disease b) Increase Milk productivity
    c) Both d) None
45. At What percentage of its live weight a buffalo consume?
    a) 2.5-3% b) 1.5- 2%
    c) 3.5-4% d) None
46. How many grazing periods occur in sheep? (10 hr per day)
    a) 3-4 times daily b) 4-7times daily
    c) 5-6 times daily d) 5-8 times daily
47. What is the average distance of movement in sheep?
    a) 8 to 16 km/ day b) 2 to 12 km/ day
    c) 5 to 10 km/day d) None
48. What are the factor which affect the amount of water ?
    a) Animal age b) Type of food
    c) Vocalization d) All
49. How many times a sheep urinate per day?
    a) 9- 13 times/ day b) 10-15 times / day
    c) 12-18 times/day d) None
50. Which animal have 3 set of gland not found in other ruminant?
    a) Sheep b) Goat
    c) Both d) None
51. New born pups do not lack the sense of?
    a) Vision b) Hearing
    c) Smell d) Touch
52. Newborn pups depend on their mother for?
    a) Food b) Elimination of body wastes
    c) Warmth d) All of the above
53. Best time for introduction of pups to human contact is?
    a) 6-8th week b) 1-2nd week
    c) 3-4th week d) 10-12th week
54. Time of sexual maturity in male dogs?
    a) 7-8 months b) 11-12 months
    c) 4-5 months d) 12-14 months

55. Time of sexual maturity In female dogs?
    a) 6-9 months b) 12-15 months
    c) 4-6 months d) 15-18 months
56. Pups gain full vision at what age?
    a) 2nd week b) 6th week
    c) 4th week d) 8th week
57. Most powerful means of communication in dogs is?
    a) Vision b) Hearing
    c) Smell d) Touch
58. Scrapping done by dogs is a method of?
    a) Aggression b) Cleaning
    c) Play d) Scent marking
59. Scrapping is commonly done by?
    a) Male dogs b) Female dogs
    c) Both a and b d) Cats
60. Which sound of dogs indicates warning of intruders or threat?
    a) Barking b) Growling
    c) Whining d) Howling
61. Which sound of dogs is the most common?
    a) Barking b) Growling
    c) Whining d) Howling
62. Which sound of dogs is an intergroup sound in the pack?
    a) Barking b) Growling
    c) Whining d) Howling
63. Which sound of dogs indicates aggression and impeding attack?
    a) Barking b) Growling
    c) Whining d) Howling
64. Which sound of dogs indicates begging for protection/attention?
    a) Barking b) Growling
    c) Whining d) Howling
65. In dogs, ears held back flat against head indicates?
    a) Submission b) Fear
    c) Aggression d) Both a and b
66. In dogs, erect ears indicate?
    a) Alertness b) Aggression
    c) Friendliness d) Both a and b
67. In dogs, tail held between legs indicate?
    a) Alertness b) Aggression
    c) Submission d) Both a and b

68. In dogs, crouching posture indicates?
   a) Alertness b) Aggression
   c) Submission d) Both a and b
69. In dogs, wagging of tail indicates?
   a) Excitement b) Aggression
   c) Submission d) Both a and b
70. In cats, wagging of tail indicates?
   a) Excitement b) Frustration
   c) Submission d) Both a and b
71. In dogs, raised hair on back, neck and shoulders indicate?
   a) Excitement b) Aggression
   c) Submission d) Both a and b
72. Play bow is shown by which animal?
   a) Dogs b) Cats
   c) Foals d) Kids
73. Mock fight in dogs indicate?
   a) Playful behavior b) Aggression
   c) Marking territory d) Mating behavior
74. Type of aggression in dogs in which male dogs attack other males but not females?
   a) Intermale aggression b) Controlled aggression
   c) Dog fight d) Territorial aggression
75. Type of aggression in dogs which is essential for training program?
   a) Intermale aggression b) Controlled aggression
   c) Spontaneous aggression d) Territorial aggression
76. Separation anxiety in dogs is displayed by?
   a) Destruction b) Excitement on return
   c) Whining d) All of the above
77. Social dominance is seen in which animals?
   a) Dogs b) Sheep
   c) Cats d) Both a and b
78. Pre- mature maternal behavior in ewes?
   a) Imprinting b) Lamb stealing
   c) Lambing d) All of the above
79. Sleeping time decreases in cattle by?
   a) Increase in roughage diet b) Decrease in roughage diet
   c) Increase in concentrate d) Both a and c
80. Cat kneading signifies?
   a) Anger b) Love and comfort
   c) Laziness d) Excitement

81. The sense of hearing is?
   a) Better in dogs than cat
   b) Better in cats than dogs
   c) Both have equal sense of hearing
   d) None of the above
82. Kittens develop sense of vision at what age?
   a) 1 week
   b) 6 weeks
   c) 3 weeks
   d) 8 weeks
83. Detection of color is better in which animal?
   a) Cats
   b) Dogs
   c) Both have equal
   d) None of the above
84. Tactile receptors in cats are present on?
   a) Paws
   b) Nose pad
   c) Whiskers
   d) All of the above
85. Most acute touch sensors in cats are?
   a) Paws
   b) Nose pad
   c) Vibrissae
   d) Both a and b
86. Forward directed whiskers indicate?
   a) Excitement
   b) Aggression
   c) Submission
   d) Fear
87. Backward directed whiskers indicate?
   a) Excitement
   b) Aggression
   c) Submission
   d) Fear
88. Hearing range of cats?
   a) 20Hz-40KHz
   b) 48Hz-85KHz
   c) 67Hz-45KHz
   d) 85Hz-100KHz
89. Hearing range of dogs?
   a) 20Hz-40KHz
   b) 48Hz-85KHz
   c) 67Hz-45KHz
   d) 85Hz-100KHz
90. Which of the following is an example of an innate behaviour in animals?
   a) Birdsong learning in songbirds
   b) Dog obedience training
   c) Nest building in birds
   d) Human language acquisition
91. What is the term for the biological rhythm that follows a roughly 24-hour cycle, affecting an animal's sleep-wake pattern and other physiological processes?
   a) Circadian rhythm
   b) Ultradian rhythm
   c) Lunar rhythm
   d) Seasonal rhythm
92. Which of the following is a behaviour that helps an animal establish dominance in a social hierarchy?
   a) Submissive behaviour
   c) Aggressive behaviour
   b) Solitary behaviour
   d) Territorial behaviour

93. When restraining an animal for medical examination or treatment, which behavior is often an indication of stress or discomfort in the animal?
   a) Eagerly following commands without resistance accepting restraint
   b) Vocalizations such as growling behavior
   c) Quietly and calmly
   d) Playful and energetic
94. What is the primary form of communication for dogs?
   a) Barking b) Whistling
   c) Meowing d) Body language
95. Why might a dog exhibit destructive behavior, such as chewing furniture or shoes?
   a) To assert dominance b) To seek attention
   c) Out of boredom or anxiety d) To show affection
96. In dog training, what is positive reinforcement?
   a) Punishing undesirable behavior
   b) Rewarding desirable behavior
   c) Ignoring undesirable behavior
   d) Using physical force to control behavior
97. When a dog exposes its belly and throat, what does this typically indicate?
   a) Submissiveness b) Playfulness
   c) Aggression d) Hunger
98. What is the recommended way to introduce two unfamiliar dogs to each other?
   a) Place them in a confined space
   b) Allow them to approach slowly and sniff
   c) Keep them on a tight leash and force to interact
   d) Keep them separated at all times
99. Which of the following body language signs indicate that a dog is becoming agitated or stressed while being restrained?
   a) Wagging tail b) Lip licking and yawning
   c) Ears forward d) Steady, relaxed breathing
100. When restraining a dog, it's important to?
   a) Approach quickly to establish dominance
   b) Speak loudly to assert authority
   c) Make direct eye contact to assert control
   d) Use calm, slow movements to avoid agitating
101. Which of the following statement is true regarding the handling of animals during feeding?
   a) Animals do not need any space during feeding
   b) The food should be spread across the entire enclosure to encourage natural foraging

c) The food should be presented on a raised platform to make it harder for animal to access

d) The caretaker should stand directly over the animal while it is eating

102. Whether the statement- It is acceptable to hit an animal if it is misbehaving.

a) True
b) Neither true or false
c) False
d) Both

103. An animal's feeding schedule can be changed abruptly without any negative consequences, this statement is-

a) True
b) Neither true or false
c) False
d) Both

104. When restraining an animal, what is the best approach to minimize stress?

a) Use the most forceful restraint possible to get the job done quickly
b) Use a familiar handler and approach slowly and calmly
c) Approach the animal quickly and loudly to establish dominance
d) Use a strong chemical tranquilizer to prevent any resistance

105. It is okay to share food with animals as long as it is not harmful to their health- this statement is -

a) True
b) Neither true or false
c) False
d) Both

106. Whether the statement is - Restraining an animal for an extended period of time can lead to stress and injury.

a) True
b) Neither true or false
c) False
d) Both

107. Restraint equipment is always necessary when handling animals- this statement is

a) True
b) Neither true or false
c) False
d) Both

108. Offering a wide variety of food options is not important for an animal's well-being.

a) True
b) Neither true or false
c) False
d) Both

109. Pulling an animal's tail or ears is a safe way to gain control of them.

a) True
b) Neither true or false
c) False
d) Both

110. Letting an animal roam free in an area with hazards is acceptable as long as it is supervised.

a) True
b) Neither true or false
c) False
d) Both

111. It is not necessary to clean feeding and watering equipment daily.

a) True
b) Neither true or false
c) False
d) Both

112. Providing ample space for an animal to move around is crucial for their physical and mental well-being.
   a) True
   b) Neither true or false
   c) False
   d) Both

113. Which of the following is a common mistake when handling animals?
   a) Not using gloves or other protective equipment
   b) Providing too much food, leading to obesity
   c) Restraining the animal too gently, allowing it to struggle
   d) Not providing any environmental enrichment

114. What is a sign of stress in animals ?
   a) lack of appetite
   c) Decreased aggression
   b) Increased activity
   d) Increased vocalization

115. What is the purpose of environmental enrichment?
   a) To give the animal things to play with
   b) To mimic the animals natural environment
   c) To keep the animal distracted so it is easier to handle
   d) To provide comfort to the animal

116. Which of the following techniques is considered aversive and should be avoided during animal restraint ?
   a) Applying pressure on the eyes
   b) Administering a local anesthetic
   c) Avoiding eye contact
   d) Placing fingers in corner of mouth

117. Which of the following statements is true regarding the appropriate way to restrain a rabbit?
   a) Grasping the loose skin over the back of the neck and lifting the rabbit by this skin is safe and humane
   b) Restrain using a towel and scruffing is only appropriate for aggressive or fractious rabbits
   c) The use of a head holder is highly recommended for safe restrain of rabbits in order to prevent struggling
   d) Rabbits should never be restrained as it is very stressful for them

118. Which of the following actions would be considered inappropriate handling of a ruminant?
   a) Administering any medical procedures without securing the head of the animal first
   c) Hugging and petting the animal before administering any medical procedures
   b) Wearing high heeled shoes when working with the animal
   d) Wrapping a rope around the neck of the animal to lead it around the enclosure

119. During feeding which of the following actions would be considered unacceptable?
   a) Feeding the animal treats in order to facilitate handling or training
   b) Offering a large amount of food at the same time so that the animal can eat as much as it wants
   c) Feeding grains that have been contaminated with mycotoxins that can harm animals
   d) Sudden introduction of a new type of food to the animals diet

120. What is the correct way to handle newborn piglets ?
   a) By the ears since piglets are born equipment with a thick auricular cartilage that minimize protects their ears from damage
   b) By the hind legs to minimize the potentially harmful kicking reflex
   c) Using specially designed snare to avoid harming the animal and struggling
   d) By the back of the neck using hand to grasp the front and heels of the piglet

121. Which of the following techniques can be used to help an animal cope with present stressors?
   a) Avoiding any interaction with the animal to avoid overwhelming it.
   b) Administering a sedative or tranquilizer to calm the animal down.
   c) Rapidly introducing it to a new and Stimulating environment to distract it.
   d) Providing the animal with an Opportunity to flee or escape its current environment.

122. Restricting an animal food and water intake can be a form of animal abuse – statement is true or false ?
   a) True b) Neither true or false
   c) False d) Both

123. It is safe to feed an animal from your hand without any previous training or acclimation – true or false?
   a) True b) Neither true or false
   c) False d) Both

124. Using punishment as a way to correct an animal's feeding behavior is an effective training technique- true or false?
   a) True b) Neither true or false
   c) False d) Both

125. It is acceptable to withhold food or water as punishment for an animal's misbehavior- true or false?
   a) True b) Neither true or false
   c) False d) Both

126. It is recommended to use positive reinforcement to encourage good feeding behavior in animals- true or false?
   a) True c) False
   b) Neither true or false d) Both

127. Which of the following should be avoided when restraining an animal?
   a) Hitting and kicking the animal body parts
   b) All of the above are acceptable
   c) Holding sensitive or painful of the animal unnecessarily
   d) Restricting the animal's air supply
128. Which of the following can you do to ensure the safety of yourself and the animal when restraining the animal?
   a) Use a proper restraint device or equipment
   b) Feed the animal while restraining
   c) Hold the animal with your bare hands
   d) Restrict the animal's air supply
129. Is it okay to feed animals with food that is not meant for their consumption?
   a) Yes
   b) Sometimes
   c) No
   d) Only on special occasions
130. Which of the following is an appropriate way to restrain an animal?
   a) Yell at the animal
   b) Hold the animal by its legs
   c) Hold the animal by its tail
   d) Use a proper restraint device or equipment
131. Which of the following should be done when trying to feed an animal?
   a) Hit the animal
   b) Approach the animal quickly and suddenly
   c) Yell at the animal
   d) Approach the animal slowly and calmly
132. Which of the following actions would be considered best practice when feeding a group of animals in a mixed species enclosure?
   a) Provide an equal amount of food to each animal in the space.
   b) Provide feeding spaces for each individual animal so that they can eat separately.
   c) Feed only one species of animal in each area to prevent competition.
   d) Feed the animals at different times of the day so that they can eat in peace.
133. Which of the following actions would be considered best practice when administering medication to a large animal?
   a) Pull the animal's tongue out of its mouth to facilitate administration.
   b) Use a syringe without a needle and administer the medication quickly, but with care.
   c) Slap the animal on the back prior to administering the medication to distract it.
   d) Hide the medication in its food or water supply to facilitate administration.

134. What is the recommended wait time after feeding an animal before handling or exercising it?

a) 1 hour
b) 5 minutes
c) 30 minutes
d) 10 minutes

135. When restraining a large animal, such as a horse or cow, what is the best way to avoid personal injury while carrying out the task?

a) Stand in front of the animal so that you can anticipate its movements and react accordingly.
b) Employ a second person when necessary and both parties stay alert and react to each other's movements.
c) Wiggle the tail of the animal to encourage it to run off, avoiding a confrontation altogether.
d) Keep as close to the animal as possible so that it feels less tempted to kick or move.

136. Providing ample space for an animal to move around is crucial for their physical and mental well-being- statement is true or false?

a) True
b) Neither true or false
c) False
d) Both

137. It is not necessary to clean feeding and watering equipment daily.

a) True
b) Neither true or false
c) False
d) Both

138. Letting an animal roam free in an area with hazards is acceptable as long as it is supervised.

a) True
b) Neither true or false
c) False
d) Both

139. Restraining an animal for an extended period of time can lead to stress and injury

a) True
b) Neither true or false
c) False
d) Both

140. Pulling an animal's tail or ears is a safe way to gain control of them.

a) True
b) Neither true or false
c) False
d) Both

141. It is okay to share food with animals as long as it is not harmful to their health

a) True
b) Neither true or false
c) False
d) Both

142. Offering a wide variety of food options is not important for an animal's well-being

a) True
b) Neither true or false
c) False
d) Both

143. An animal's feeding schedule can be changed abruptly without any negative consequences?

a) True
b) Neither true or false
c) False
d) Both

144. Restraint equipment is always necessary when handling animals?
   a) True b) Neither true or false
   c) False d) Both
145. It is acceptable to hit an animal if it is misbehaving- true or false?
   a) True b) Neither true or false
   c) False d) Both
146. What is the primary reason for cattle exhibiting social grooming behavior?
   a) Maintaining hygiene b) Establishing dominance
   c) Communication d) Seeking attention
147. What is a common behavior exhibited by cattle in a herd?
   a) Solitary grazing b) Nocturnal activity
   c) Aggressive dominance d) Herbivore hunting
148. What is a common behavior exhibited by pigs when they are content and relaxed?
   a) Aggressive grunting b) Constant pacing
   c) Tail wagging d) Loud squealing
149. What is a common behavior exhibited by goats when they are excited or playful?
   a) Wagging their tails b) Bleating loudly
   c) Standing still d) Avoiding eye contact
150. What does it generally mean when a horse lays its ears back flat against its head?
   a) Contentment b) Excitement
   c) Aggression or irritation d) Fear

Answer Key

1	c	2	b	3	a	4	b	5	b	6	a	7	d
8	a	9	a	10	b	11	c	12	b	13	d	14	d
15	a	16	b	17	a	18	c	19	a	20	b	21	b
22	b	23	a	24	a	25	b	26	a	27	d	28	d
29	b	30	a	31	b	32	d	33	a	34	c	35	d
36	a	37	b	38	a	39	b	40	b	41	c	42	b
43	a	44	c	45	a	46	c	47	a	48	d	49	a
50	a	51	d	52	d	53	a	54	a	55	a	56	c
57	c	58	d	59	a	60	a	61	a	62	d	63	b
64	c	65	d	66	d	67	c	68	c	69	c	70	b
71	b	72	a	73	a	74	a	75	b	76	d	77	d
78	b	79	a	80	b	81	b	82	c	83	a	84	d
85	c	86	b	87	d	88	b	89	c	90	c	91	a
92	c	93	b	94	d	95	b	96	b	97	a	98	b
99	b	100	d	101	b	102	d	103	d	104	b	105	d
106	c	107	a	108	c	109	c	110	a	111	c	112	a
113	a	114	a	115	c	116	d	117	d	118	c	119	d

120	d	121	a	122	a	123	d	124	c	125	c	126	a
127	b	128	a	129	c	130	d	131	d	132	c	133	d
134	c	135	c	136	d	137	c	138	c	139	a	140	c
141	a	142	c	143	c	144	a	145	b	146	a	147	c
148	c	149	b	150	c								

3

Behaviour in Host-Parasite Interaction

Sirigireddy Sivajothi[1], Bhavanam Sudhakara Reddy[1] and Tanmoy Rana[2]

[1]NTR College of Veterinary Science - Gannavaram, Sri Venkateswara Veterinary University, Andhra Pradesh

[2]Department of Veterinary Clinical Complex, West Bengal University of Animal & Fishery Sciences, Kolkata, West Bengal

Introduction

In a host-parasite relationship, the interaction between the two organisms is highly specialized. Each partner impacts the other's life by influencing their metabolism and behavior through various adaptive mechanisms, all aimed at ensuring their own survival. While the parasite exerts every effort to fully establish itself within the host—by consuming its resources, damaging its tissues, secreting toxins, and evading the host's immune system through molecular mimicry—the host, in turn, strives to eliminate the parasite by mobilizing its immune defenses.

Despite their ongoing conflict, neither the host nor the parasite is able to completely eradicate the other. The host seeks to fend off the harmful, invasive parasite, while the parasite aims to establish a lasting, close relationship with the host. However, this dynamic can lead to a point where either the host or the parasite, often the parasite, becomes dominant or independent, resulting in the death of one party. Thus, the host-parasite relationship appears to be a perpetual and interdependent one, each partner intricately tied to the other.

When a parasite enters a host, the host must make adjustments, and the parasite must adapt to the host's environment. This interaction leads to the development of a relationship in which both the host and the parasite influence each other's growth, metabolism, and overall well-being. Generally, the host-parasite relationship unfolds through a series of stages: it starts with the transmission of the parasite from one host to another, followed by the parasite's distribution and localization within or on the new host. This is followed by the parasite's growth or multiplication. Throughout this process, both the host and the parasite engage in resistance efforts against each other.

The process involves several stages: the parasite's method of attack, the changes the parasite induces in the host, and the alterations the parasite undergoes due to its presence in the host. It also includes the adjustments made by both host and parasite during the infection, the escape of the parasite's infective stages from the host, and ultimately, the host's recovery or death.

In the host-parasite relationship, there are two main categories of bio-physiological functions: 1. Parasite invasiveness, which focuses on gaining entry into the host and sustaining life within it, and 2. Host resistance, which aims to prevent the parasite's invasion and colonization.

In a host-parasite relationship, these functions act in opposition, maintaining a balance between the two entities. As the parasite grows and multiplies within or on the host, the host is considered to be infected.

Since parasitic organisms are, by definition, dependent on their hosts, the symbiotic relationship between the host and parasite can be described as follows:

Mutualism
Commensalism
Parasitism

Another intriguing and challenging aspect of the host-parasite relationship is the impact of the parasite on the host's biology.

Among the most significant and fascinating effects are the secondary manifestations that result from damage to specific organs. For example, crabs parasitized by Sacculina experience severe alterations in their genital tissues; this parasitic crustacean causes dramatic changes in the males, but not in the females. In 70% of parasitized male crabs, the testes undergo degeneration, and the crabs develop secondary female characteristics. Similarly, parasitized female crabs experience changes in their ovarian tissue, leading to the acquisition of male characteristics. Consequently, there is a complete loss of sexual dimorphism in these infected crabs.

However, if the parasites are removed, the female crabs' ovaries return to their normal state, while the males' previously atrophied testes develop into ovotestes, which can produce both eggs and sperm. This phenomenon, where the parasite induces such changes in the host, is known as parasitic castration. The parasitic isopod *Entoniscus* initially attaches as an ectoparasite but soon enters the host's body cavity. Remarkably, it causes castration without ever directly interacting with the host's gonads.

Another intriguing biological change induced by parasites involves metabolic alterations in the host. For instance, when the ant *Pheidole commulata* is parasitized by the nematode *Mermis*, it undergoes hypertrophy, resulting in a significantly larger body size compared to normal ants.

Behaviour in Host-Parasite Interactions

MCQ's

1. For the host, the most dangerous relationship with another organism is

   a) Symbiosis b) Parasitism

   c) Commensalism d) Mutualism

2. The term ectoparasites includes

   a) Some Viruses b) Some bacteria

   c) Some Protozoans d) Some insects

3. What is a relationship between organisms of different species where an organism is benefited and other is harmed called?
   a) Symbiosis
   b) Parasitism
   c) Commensalism
   d) Mutualism
4. Where do ectoparasites reside?
   a) Within the blood
   b) In the intercellular spaces of host
   c) Within the cells
   d) On the surface of the host
5. Where do endo-parasites reside?
   a) Within the cells of the host body
   b) On the surface of the host body
   c) Outside the skin of the host
   d) Outside the host environment
6. What is an organism carrying another organism to the host called?
   a) Parasite
   b) Vector
   c) Pathogen
   d) Bacteria
7. The parasite which cannot survive without a host is known as
   a) Facultative
   b) Periodic
   c) Spurious
   d) Obligatory
8. The host which prolongs the lifecycle without any development is known as
   a) Final host
   b) Unnatural host
   c) Paratenic host
   d) Carrier host
9. Parasite having broad host range is known as
   a) Monoxenous
   b) Heteroxenous
   c) Euryxenous
   d) Stenoxenous
10. Most common class of antibody encountered in immunity to tissue helminths is
    a) IgM
    b) Ig G
    c) IgD
    d) IgE
11. A host which carry the infective stage of a parasite of another host without any development is a
    a) Definitive host
    b) Accidental host
    c) Transport host
    d) Intermediate host
12. Transformation of tissue from one type to another in response to parasite is known as
    a) Metaplasia
    b) Hyperplasia
    c) Cirrhosis
    d) Hypertrophy
13. A host which harbour the residual stage of the parasite in a latent phase is
    a) Alternate host
    b) Carrier host
    c) Intermediate host
    d) Vector

14. Relationship between two organisms wherein both the partners are benefited is
    a) Mutualism b) Parasitism
    c) Phoresy d) Commensalism
15. The endoparasites found inside the cells of the host is better known as
    a) Intercellular parasite b) Extracellular parasite
    c) Intracellular parasite d) Interstitial parasite
16. The organism parasitizing an animal which is not its definitive host is known as
    a) Aberrant parasite b) Accidental parasite
    c) Erratic parasite d) Ectopic parasite
17. A host which harbours the larval or asexual stage and is vital for completion of parasite's lifecycle is called
    a) Intermediate host b) Definitive host
    c) Aberrant host d) Transport host
18. The parasite which does not absolutely depend on parasitic life but had a period of free existence
    a) Obligatory b) Free living
    c) Facultative d) Mutualism
19. The parasite which live only on one type of host during the course of their life is called a
    a) Monoxenous b) Euryxenous
    c) Heteroxenous d) Stenoxenous
20. The parasites which live in two or more types of hosts during the course of their life are called
    a) Monoxenous b) Homoxenous
    c) Heteroxenous d) Stenoxenous
21. Parasite with a narrow hot range is called
    a) Monoxenous b) Homoxenous
    c) Heteroxenous d) Stenoxenous
22. The parasite that lives within the tissues of the host is known as
    a) Histozoic parasite b) Coelozoic parasite
    c) Histotrophic parasite d) Ectoparasite
23. The parasite which lays eggs is known as
    a) Oviparous b) Ovo-viviparous
    c) Viviparous d) Pupiparous
24. The parasite which lays eggs containing fully developed larvae is knowns
    a) Oviparous b) Ovo-viviparous
    c) Viviparous d) Pupiparous
25. The female parasite which lays larvae is known as
    a) Oviparous b) Ovo-viviparous
    c) Viviparous d) Pupiparous

26. The parasite which lays pupa is known as
    a) Oviparous
    b) Ovo-viviparous
    c) Viviparous
    d) Pupiparous
27. A host that has a residual population of parasites and which acts as a source of infection for the same type of hosts is known as
    a) Definitive host
    b) Reservoir host
    c) Carrier host
    d) Paratenic host
28. The host which harbors the sexual stage of a parasite is known as
    a) Definitive host
    b) Reservoir host
    c) Carrier host
    d) Intermediate host
29. The host which harbors the adult stage of a parasite is known as
    a) Definitive host
    b) Reservoir host
    c) Carrier host
    d) Intermediate host
30. The host which harbors the larval stage of a parasite is known as
    a) Definitive host
    b) Reservoir host
    c) Carrier host
    d) Intermediate host
31. The following a vertebrate host in which a parasite occurs naturally without producing any harm to the host
    a) Definitive host
    b) Reservoir host
    c) Carrier host
    d) Intermediate host
32. The host which harbours the sexually mature parasite of another definitive host and acts as source of infection to the original definitive host is known as
    a) Definitive host
    b) Reservoir host
    c) Carrier host
    d) Intermediate host
33. In which of the following types of hosts, the parasite gets encapsulated in the tissues without any further development
    a) Definitive host
    b) Reservoir host
    c) Paratenic host
    d) Intermediate host
34. The vector in which the parasite does not develop or multiply but simply is transmitted is known as
    a) Biological
    b) Cyclical
    c) Mechanical
    d) Vertical
35. The host which harbours residual parasite in a latent phase without showing clinical symptoms of a disease is called as
    a) Definitive host
    b) Reservoir host
    c) Paratenic host
    d) Carrier hot
36. The intracellular haemoprotozoan which causes intravascular haemolysis leading to progressive anaemia, haemoglobinuria, jaundice & its piroplasms are observed inside the RBC is
    a) Babesia spp
    b) Ehrlichia sps
    c) Trypanosoma cruzi
    d) None

37. Parasitism is a state in which the parasite is dependent on the host for the following
    a) Physiologically b) Pathologically
    c) Biologically d) Metabolically
38. The host-parasite relationship that best describes eating at the common table is describes as
    a) Commensalism b) Ammensalism
    c) Phoresis d) Symbiosis
39. In which of the following relationships, one organism receives some benefits while the other neither gets benefited nor harmed
    a) Commensalism b) Mutualism
    c) Phoresis d) Symbiosis
40. The term used to describe a host that is typically suited for complete development of a particular parasite is known as
    a) Normal host/usual hot b) Reservoir host
    c) Abnormal host/ unusual host d) Carrier hot
41. The association in which parasite injures the host and produces pathological lesion is known as
    a) Parasitosis b) Infection
    c) Parasitoids d) Infestation
42. The following relationship is obligatory and permanent
    a) Symbiosis b) Phoresis
    c) Mutualism d) Commensalism
43. The parasite-host relationship that literally describes 'travelling together' is
    a) Symbiosis b) Phoresis
    c) Mutualism d) Commensalism
44. In the following type of relationship, there will be no metabolic dependance
    a) Symbiosis b) Phoresis
    c) Mutualism d) Commensalism
45. The following is the synonym of co-infectious immunity
    a) Premunity b) Concominant immunity
    c) Solid immunity d) Sterile immunity
46. Biotic potential refers to the following
    a) Fecundity b) Mortality
    c) Morbidity d) Fatality
47. The following is often referred to as micropredator
    a) Permanent parasite b) Temporary parasite
    c) Obligatory parasite d) Facultative parasite
48. The process of transformation of cysts to trophozoite when it enters into alimentary canal of susceptible host is termed as
    a) Excystation b) Encystation
    c) Sporulation d) Predation

49. The following cell is capable of killing host cell infected with intracellular Parasite
    a) CD4 helper T-cell b) CD8 cytotoxic T-cell
    c) Mast cell d) Lymphocyte
50. Feeding of colostrum to young ones is an example of which type of immunity
    a) Active b) Passive
    c) Innate d) Natural
51. Which type of immunoglobulin is immunodominant in helminthic infection
    a) IgG b) IgM
    c) IgA d) IgE
52. Eosinophilia is the major characteristic feature in which type of infection
    a) Helminth b) Arthropod
    c) Protozoa d) Ticks and Mites
53. *Trypanosoma cruzi* escapes the immune system of host by the following mechanism
    a) Prevents fusion of phagosome with lysosome
    b) Escapes into cytosol
    c) Resistance to lysosomal enzymes
    d) Shedding of antigens
54. What are the molecular tools used for identification of a parasite gene
    a) Microarray b) RNA interference
    c) Phage display d) All of the above
55. The parasite evades the host immune responses by the following mechanisms
    a) Antigenic variation b) Antigenic disguise
    c) Antigenic mimicry d) All of the above
56. Level of which of the following immunoglobulins are raised in visceral leishmaniosis and malaria
    a) IgG b) IgM
    c) IgA d) IgE
57. Ig A I the predominant immunoglobulin found in
    a) Blood b) Tissue
    c) Secretions d) Skin
58. Cell-mediated immune response requires the following
    a) B-cell activation b) Macrophage activation
    c) T-cell activation d) All the above
59. Which form of immunity lacks any form of memory, and each infection is treated identically
    a) Acquired immunity b) Preimmunity
    c) Concomitant immunity d) Innate immunity
60. In general cell mediated immune responses are more effective against
    a) Intracellular protozoa b) Extracellular protozoa
    c) Intestinal protozoa d) Ruminal protozoa

61. Dogs act as ______ in the life cycle of Sarcocystis
   a) Intermediate host   b) Definitive host
   c) Paratenic host   d) None of the above
62. The following are the zoonotic protozoan parasites of dogs & cats
   a) Sarcocystis   b) Toxoplasma gondii
   c) Cryptosporidium   d) All the above
63. Mange infestation is mediated by
   a) Immediate hypersensitive reaction
   b) Cytotoxic hypersensitive reaction
   c) Immune complex hypersensitive reaction
   d) Delayed type hypersensitive reaction
64. The type of hypersensitivity mediated in self cure phenomenon is
   a) Type I   b) Type II
   c) Type III   d) Type IV
65. A suspension of living or inactivated organisms used as an antigen to confer immunity
   a) Culture   b) Vaccine
   c) Media   d) Passage
66. The immunoglobulin involved in immediate type I hypersensitive reaction when bound to mast cells
   a) IgM   b) IgE
   c) IgE   d) IgA
67. Antigenic variation in trypanosomosis is due
   a) VSG   b) Mucoproteins
   c) Glycopolysaccharides   d) Integument
68. Dogs showing pancytopenia, oedema of limbs, lymphadenopathy monocytosis and epistaxis may be infected with
   a) Ehrlichia canis   b) Heptozoon canis
   c) Sacrocystis cruzi   d) Toxoplasma gondii
69. Lung fluke of Cat is
   a) Paragonimus westermani   b) Paragonimus kellicotti
   c) Prosthogonimus ovatus   d) Paramphistomum cervi
70. Hypersensitivity test used in diagnosis of Echinococcosis in Humans
   a) Montenergo intradermal skin test
   b) Brucellin test
   c) Tuberculin test
   d) Casonils intradermal skin test
71. Broad fish tape worm is
   a) Echinococcus granulosus   b) Echinococcus multilocularis
   c) Diphyllobothrium latum   d) Dipylidium caninum

72. Serum protein containing antibody activity is termed as
   a) Opsonin b) Immunoglobulin
   c) Antitoxin d) Hapten
73. Fish eating mammals can be infected by
   a) Echinococcus granulosus b) Echinococcus multilocularis
   c) Diphyllobothrium latum d) Dipylidium caninum
74. Immunocompromised individual can be infected with
   a) Cryptosporidium parva b) Echinococcus granulosus
   c) Eimeria tenella d) Isospora felis
75. Infective stage of Dipylidium caninum for dogs is
   a) Procercoid b) Pleurocercoid
   c) Coracidium d) Cysticercoid
76. Definitive host for Dipylidium caninum
   a) Cattle b) Dog
   c) Sheep d) Goats
77. Intermediate host for Dipylidium caninum
   a) Fleas b) Lice
   c) Both a & b d) Ticks
78. Infective stage of Diphyllobothrium latum for dogs is
   a) Procercoid b) Pleurocercoid
   c) Coracidium d) Cysticercoid
79. Prenatal transmission is absent in
   a) Toxocara canis b) Toxocara cati
   c) Toxocaris leonina d) Both b & c
80. Transmammary route of transmission is seen in
   a) Toxocara canis b) Toxocara cati
   c) Toxocaris leonine d) Both b & c
81. Visceral larva migrans is caused by
   a) Toxocara sps b) Schistosoma sps
   c) Ancyclostoma sps d) None
82. Oesophageal tumor worm of dogs is
   a) Gongylonema pulchrum b) Spirocerca lupi
   c) Physalopteria praeputialis d) None
83. Physaloptera praeputialis is also known as
   a) Stomach worm of cat b) Heart worm of Dog
   c) Gullet worm of Dogs d) Eye worm of Dog
84. Following nematode is known as the "Stomach worms of Dogs & cats" which has a zoonotic importance with man as the 2nd intermediate host
   a) Gongylonema pulchrum b) Physaloptera preputalis
   c) Gnathostoma spinigerum d) Gongylonema ingluvicola

85. Paratenic host for Toxocara canis
 a) Cat b) Rodents
 c) Dogs d) Cattle

86. Predilictron site for immature larvae of spirocera lupi
 a) Oesophagus b) Stomach
 c) Liver d) Aorta

87. Stenosis of aorta& hypertrophic osteopathy of long bones are the complications of ________________ infection
 a) Dirofilaria immitis b) Spirocerca lupi
 c) Gnathostoma spinigerum d) None of the above

88. Reddish spirally coiled worms present as nodules in the oesophagus of dogs is:
 a) Gnathostoma sps b) Dirofilaria sps
 c) Spirocera lupi d) Gongylonema pulchrum

89. Intermediate host for spirocera lupi is
 a) Sheep b) Coprophagus beetles
 c) Cyprinid fish d) Cyclops

90. Intermediate host for Dirofilaria immitis is
 a) Anopheles mosquitoes b) Culicine mosquitoes
 c) Tabanid files d) Cyclops

91. The endosymbiotic bacteria thet lives intacellularly in dirofilaria immitis is
 a) Clostridium novyi b) Fusobacterium
 c) Bacteriodus nodosus d) Wolbachia pipiens

92. Diagnosis of canine heart worm can be done by
 a) Microfilaria demonstration b) ECG
 c) Chest radiography d) All of the above

93. The larval stage of dirofilaria immitis (L1) is called as
 a) Hydatid cyst b) Procercoid
 c) Microfilaria d) Coenurus

94. Masses of heart worms in the posterior vena cava with symptoms of icterus, haemoglobinuria, haemoptysis, hepatic dysfunction leading to a condition called as
 a) Endocarditis b) Nairobi bleeding diseas
 c) Vena caval syndrome d) None of the above

95. Dogs with list lessness, loss of condition, chronic soft cough, Endocarditis and presence of microfilaria in peripheral blood are infected with
 a) Spirocera lupi b) Parafilaraia multipapillosus
 c) Both a & b d) Dirofilaria immitis

96. Prediliction sites of Dirofilaria immitis are:
 a) Right ventricle b) Pulmonary artery
 c) Posterior venacava d) All of the above

97. Infective stage of dirofilaria immits for intermediate host is
    a) L2 Larva b) Eggs
    c) L3 Larva d) Microfilaria
98. Strongyloides Papillosus is parasite of
    a) Sheep b) Goat
    c) Pig d) Dog
99. Stephanurus dentatus is parasite of
    a) Shee b) Goat
    c) Pig d) Dog
100. Bloood sucking stage of ancylostoma canium is
    a) Adult Worms b) L3
    c) L4 d) L5
101. Dogs with tarry coloured faeces, anemia & presence of 8-celled Strongyle egg is infected with
    a) Ancylostoma caninum b) Strongylus vulgaris
    c) Strongylus edentates d) Both b & c
102. Cutaneous larva migrans is caused by larvae of
    a) Toxocara canis b) Toxocara cati
    c) Schistosoma nasale d) Ancyclostomum caninum
103. Ancyclostomum caninum worms suck upto _______ ml of Blood per day
    a) 0.1ml b) 0.01ml
    c) 0.001ml d) 0.0001ml
104. Canine hook worm vaccine contains
    a) Inactivated L1 b) Stomach protein Antigen
    c) Irradiated L3 larvae d) None
105. Miller vaccine is against
    a) Strongylus vulgaris b) Ancyclostomum canium
    c) Bunostomum trigonocephalum d) Stephanofilaria assamensis
106. Immunological phenomenon called CRISIS occurs in the following parasite
    a) Ancyclostoma canium b) Toxocara canis
    c) Spirocera lupi d) All of the above
107. The following parasite is known as lung worm of dog
    a) Dictyocaulus viviparous b) Filaroides osleri
    c) Dictyocaulus filaria d) Spirocera lupi
108. Aelurostrongylus abstrusus is commonly known as
    a) Lung worm of cattle b) Lung worm of Sheep & Goat
    c) Eye worm of Dog d) Lung worm of Cat

109. Tear drop shaped protozoan parasite with 8 flagella which causes steatorrhoea in man & dog is

a) Leshmania tropica
b) Trypanosoma cruzi
c) Giardia canis
d) None of the above

110. Paratenic host of Spirocera lupi is

a) Garden lizard (calotes)
b) Chicken
c) Both a & b
d) None of the above

111. The scolex of Diphyllobothorium latum is

a) Armed
b) Almond shaped
c) Oval
d) Spherical

112. Whip worm of canines is

a) Trichuris ovis
b) Trichuris suis
c) Trichuris globose
d) Trichuris vulpis

113. Location of Trichories vulpis is

a) Stomach
b) Small intestine
c) Caecum & Colon
d) Skin

114. Location of Toxoplasma gondii in cats

a) Small intestine
b) Stomach
c) Oesophagus
d) Lungs

115. Mode of transmission of Taxoplasma gondii is

a) Congential
b) Carnivorism
c) Oro-faecal route
d) All of the above

116. The definitive of host of Neospora canium is

a) Dogs
b) Cattle
c) Sheep & Goat
d) Pigs

117. The parasite infections of dogs caused by ingestion of row offals /uncooked meat are

a) Sarcocystosis
b) Echinococcosis
c) Neosporosis
d) All of the above

118. Asexual stages of Hepatozoon canis are present in

a) Definative host
b) Intermediate host
c) Paratenic host
d) Environment

119. The groups of Ehrlichia canis organisms inside the monocytes are termed as

a) Morula
b) Piroplasms
c) Amastigote
d) Promastigote

120. The following is the rickettsial pathogen of cats

a) Ehrlichia canis
b) Haemobartonella
c) Anaplasma centrale
d) All of the above

121. The parasite commonly known as " Oriental Lung Fluke" is
   a) Paragonimus westermanii b) Taenia saginata
   c) Opisthorchris tenuicollis d) Clonorchis sinensis
122. "Chinese liver fluke" of Dog & Cat is
   a) Paragonimus westermanii b) Clonorchis sinensis
   c) Opisthorchis tenuicollis d) Taenia saginata
123. Type of anemia seen in Ancyclostomiosis is
   a) Macrocytic hypochromic b) Microcytic hypochromic
   c) Normocytic normochromic d) All of the above
124. Type of anemia seen in Diphyllobothriosis is
   a) Normocytic normochromic b) Microcytic hypochromic
   c) Macrocytic hypochromic d) None of the above
125. Fish borne termatode infections of Dogs & cats
   a) Opisthorchis tenuicollis b) Heterophyes heterophyes
   c) Clonorchis sinensis d) All of the above
126. Beaver fever is caused by
   a) Giardia intestinalis b) Balantidium coli
   c) Entamoeba coli d) All of the above
127. Cholangitis and hepatic carcinoma in dogs is caused by
   a) Dicrocoelium dendriticum b) Fasciola hepatica
   c) Opisthorchis tenuicollis d) Fasciolopsis buski
128. Small intestinal fluke of dogs and cats is
   a) Dicrocoelium dendriticum b) Heterophyes heterophyes
   c) Opisthorchis tenuicollis d) Paragonimus westermanii
129. Y- shaped excretory bladder is seen in the following trematode
   a) Opisthorchis tenuicollis b) Dicrocoelium dendriticum
   c) Fasciola hepatica d) Fasciola gigantica
130. Entero-epithelial cycle of Toxoplasma gondii occurs in
   a) Sheep and goat b) Cats
   c) Dogs d) Humans
131. The metacestode stage of Dipylidium caninum is
   a) Cysticercus b) Coenurus
   c) Hydatid cyst d) Cysticercoid
132. Ovary and vitelline glands of Dipylidium caninum resembles
   a) Bunch of grapes b) Cucumber seeds
   c) Dog louse d) None of the above
133. The definitive host for Taenia taeniaeformis is
   a) Dog b) Rabbit
   c) Cat d) Sheep

134. The metacestode of Taenia taeniaeformis is
   a) Coenurus b) Strobilocercus
   c) Hydatid cyst d) Cysticercoid
135. Alveolar hydatidosis in wild fox is caused by
   a) Echinococcus granulosus b) Dipylidium caninum
   c) Echinococcus multiocularis d) None of the above
136. Hydatid cysts without protoscolices and are therefore not infective to dogs are called as
   a) Sterile cysts b) Fertile cysts
   c) Brood capsules d) Protoscolices
137. The dog with Echinococcosis is orally purged with
   a) Metaclopromide b) Liquid paraffin
   c) Vinegar d) Arecoline hydrobromide
138. The scolex of Diphyllobothrium latum contains narrow longitudinal muscular grooves called
   a) Proglottids b) Suckers
   c) Hooks d) Bothria
139. Free- living ciliated embryo of Diphyllobothrium latum is called
   a) Procercoid b) Plerocercoid
   c) Coracidium d) None
140. Naked Sporozoites are seen in
   a) Cryptosporidium b) Neospora
   c) Toxoplasma d) Sarcocystis
141. Eggs of Diphyllobothrium latum are seen in faeces of
   a) Dogs b) Sheep
   c) Cattle d) None
142. Pressure atrophy of tissues of host is associated with
   a) Strobilocercosis b) Cystic Echinococcosis
   c) Taeniosis d) Cysticereosis
143. Creeping eruption in children in caused by
   a) Toxocara canis b) Ancyclostoma braziliensis
   c) Schistosoma nasale d) Cysticercus cellulosae
144. Leishman denovan bodies seen in which cells
   a) RBC b) Eosinophils
   c) Platelets d) Macrophages
145. Microfilaria is transmitted by
   a) Direct contact b) Ingestion
   c) Vector d) Air

146. Mode of transmission of filariasis in dogs is
   a) Ingestion of Intermediate host
   b) Inoculation by vector
   c) Inhalation of Infective stage
   d) None
147. Malignant Jaundice in dogs is caused by
   a) Babesia canis
   b) Hepatozoon canis
   c) Trypanosoma cruzi
   d) Ehrlichia canis
148. The following haematoprotozoan disease of dogs should be differentiated from rabies
   a) Babesia canis
   b) Hepatozoonosis
   c) Trypanosomosis
   d) Ehrlichiosis
149. The following disease is otherwise known as Canine Strongylosis
   a) Toxocara infection
   b) Schistosomosis
   c) Bunostomosis
   d) Ancyclostomosis
150. Oesophageal fibrosarcoma and osteosarcoma in dogs is caused by
   a) Gongylonema pulchrum
   b) Gnathostoma
   c) Spirocerca lupi
   d) Physaloptera

Answer Key

1	b	2	d	3	b	4	d	5	c	6	b	7	d
8	c	9	c	10	d	11	c	12	a	13	b	14	a
15	c	16	b	17	a	18	c	19	a	20	c	21	d
22	a	23	a	24	d	25	c	26	c	27	c	28	a
29	a	30	d	31	b	32	b	33	c	34	c	35	d
36	a	37	d	38	a	39	a	40	a	41	a	42	c
43	b	44	b	45	a	46	a	47	b	48	a	49	a
50	b	51	d	52	a	53	b	54	d	55	d	56	a
57	c	58	c	59	d	60	a	61	b	62	d	63	a
64	a	65	b	66	b	67	a	68	a	69	b	70	d
71	c	72	b	73	c	74	a	75	b	76	b	77	c
78	b	79	d	80	d	81	a	82	b	83	a	84	c
85	c	86	d	87	b	88	c	89	b	90	b	91	d
92	d	93	c	94	c	95	d	96	d	97	d	98	a
99	c	100	d	101	a	102	d	103	c	104	c	105	b
106	a	107	b	108	d	109	c	110	c	111	b	112	d
113	c	114	a	115	d	116	a	117	d	118	a	119	a
120	b	121	a	122	b	123	b	124	c	125	d	126	a
127	c	128	b	129	a	130	b	131	d	132	a	133	c
134	b	135	c	136	a	137	d	138	d	139	c	140	a
141	a	142	a	143	a	144	d	145	c	146	b	147	a
148	c	149	d	150	c								

4

Behaviour of Courtship

Jayanta Das[1], Rajesh Kumar[1], Sushant Sivastava[1] and Pramod Kumar[2]

[1]*Department of Veterinary Gynaecology and Obstetrics, College of Veterinary Science & Animal Husbandry, Acharya Narendra Deva University of Agriculture & Technology, Ayodhya, Uttar Pradesh*

[2]*Department of Veterinary Physiology and Biochemistry, College of Veterinary Science & Animal Husbandry, Acharya Narendra Deva University of Agriculture & Technology, Ayodhya, Uttar Pradesh*

Introduction

An animal will engage in a series of display activities known as courtships to try to entice a mate and show that it wants to copulate. These actions frequently take the form of vocalisations, mechanical sound production, ritualised movement (referred to as "dances"), or exhibitions of physical prowess, agonistic aptitude, or beauty. A social activity known as courtship occurs when male and female members of the same species engage in order to facilitate mating and reproduction. Because so many sperm are created and must find and fertilise a small number of eggs, sperm rivalry led to the evolution of courtship. Males must compete with one another for the female's sperm in order to fertilise her eggs, which are a finite supply. Male-to-male competition and female choice are the results of sexual selection between men and females, which is a translation of gametic selection. An offshoot of this male-male competition is the courtship display, where men have developed a variety of tools and strategies to entice females to procreate.

MCQ's

1. When an animal attempts to attract a mate and exhibit their desire to copulate, the behaviour is termed as

   a) Mount b) Courtship
   c) Flehmen reaction d) None of the above

2. Extension of the male-male competition in which males evolved various devices and techniques to persuade female to reproduce:

   a) Mount b) Courtship
   c) Flehmen reaction d) None of the above

3. Courtship refers to the behavioural interaction that occurs between males and females:
   a) During mating
   b) Before mating
   c) After mating
   d) All of the above
4. Courtship behaviour occurs between
   a) Between same species
   b) Between different species
   c) Both a & b
   d) None of the above
5. Semen is ejaculated as a single violent rush intra-vaginally near
   a) Os-cervix
   b) Ampula
   c) Uterus
   d) None of these
6. What happens to males, if one sense is inhibited?
   a) Behavior becomes more erratic
   b) Another sense is augmented
   c) All senses are equally diminished
   d) The male stops trying to copulate
7. How does sensory deprivation affect copulation in domestic mammals?
   a) It only affects inexperienced males
   b) It completely stops copulation
   c) It makes copulation totally ineffective
   d) It does not suppress copulation if contact is made
8. Which one of the following stimuli is involved in the organization of postural responses during copulation?
   a) Olfactory stimuli
   b) Visual stimuli
   c) Tactile stimuli
   d) Auditory stimuli
9. What is important for the normal development of mounting and thrusting behaviours in bulls and goats?
   a) Visual stimulation
   b) Sensory input from the penis
   c) Auditory input
   d) Olfactory cues
10. Which physiologic signal is responsible for initiating sexual motivation?
    a) Neuronal circuits
    b) Visual and tactile cues
    b) Hormonal imbalance
    d) Gonadal steroid balance
11. What occurs during the 'standing reaction' in sows?
    a) The sow lies down and remains motionless
    b) The sow becomes absolutely immobile, arches her back, and cocks her ears
    c) The sow squeals loudly and digs the ground
    d) The sow starts moving frantically and becomes restless

12. What percentage of estrous gilts will show the standing reaction if presented with the odour of a boar?
    a) 60% b) 100%
    c) 30% d) 48%
13. What is a primary trigger for a male animal's mounting behavior?
    a) The acoustic signals from the female
    b) The overall shape and immobility of the female
    c) The olfactory cues from the female
    d) The restrained condition of the female
14. Which stimuli are also likely to trigger sexual reactions in a bull or boar?
    a) The sound of a female in estrus b) A restrained male or a dummy
    c) A moving female d) The scent of food
15. Which of the following is most important in encounter of sexual partners in free-living animals?
    a) Availability of food sources
    b) Weather conditions
    c) Pre-existing social structure and territorial behavior
    d) Predation risks
16. How do male rabbits display sexual behavior in artificial environments?
    a) By responding to any nearby female rabbits immediately
    b) After adapting to the artificial environment within a few minutes
    c) When they see another male rabbit
    d) By considering the cage their territory after occupying it for a long period
17. What is the basic unit of social structure among farm animals like African antelopes and Bisons?
    a) A stable matriarchal herd
    b) A mixed group of unrelated individuals
    c) A transient group that changes frequently
    d) A solitary male
18. The social organization in ungulates are regulated by
    a) Bond between dams and their female offspring
    b) Competition for food resources
    c) Migration patterns
    d) Interaction with predators
19. The consequence of high population density in ungulates is ?
    a) Improved performance of all animals
    b) Greater bonding among ungulates
    c) Abnormal behavior such as cannibalism
    d) Decreased levels of aggression

20. What is 'tending behaviour' commonly associated with?
    a) Independent feeding behaviour
    b) Juvenile learning behaviour
    c) Male pre-copulatory behaviou
    d) Female post-copulatory behaviour
21. The "tending behaviour" among both sexes results in
    a) A temporary bonding
    b) Noise making
    c) Hunting together
    d) A permanent nest
22. What might happen if the tending male loses interest?
    a) Other bulls may replace him
    b) They build a nest
    c) The female leaves the area
    d) The male starts to feed
23. The male detect pheromones from the female via
    a) Smells the female's urine
    b) Touches the female's ears
    c) Listens to the female's sounds
    d) Eats the female's food
24. The 'Flehmen' response involve?
    a) Lying down and closing eyes
    b) Stamping feet and shaking head
    c) Running in circles and wagging tail
    d) Forward extended neck and curled upper lip
25. The flehmen behaviour related to?
    a) Auditory responses by the ears
    b) Visual sensory evaluation by the eyes
    c) Chemo-sensory evaluation by the Vomeronasal organ
    d) Digestive tract movements
26. The flehmen behaviour is rarely performed by females during
    a) While grazing at pasture
    b) When sniffing male urine
    c) In response to handler's clothing
    d) During sexual encounters with males
27. What does a male goat do to test receptivity of female goat?
    a) Licks and sniffs the female
    b) Kicks the female gently
    c) Makes loud noises
    d) Walks in circles around the female
28. What behavior do oestrous cows show when they respond to chin-resting pressure?
    a) They kick the male
    b) They moo loudly
    c) They lie down
    d) They stand stationary to be mounted

29. What behavior does a bull show when a female buffalo is in oestrus?
    a) Lays down next to her
    b) Rests his chin on her
    c) Eats from the same spot
    d) Runs around her
30. In bulls, the accessory fluid is excreted from?
    a) Pelvic gland
    b) Vesicular glands
    c) Thyroid gland
    d) Cowper's gland
31. What happens to a bull's penis during unsuccessful mounts?
    a) Becomes fully rigid
    b) Becomes partially erected
    c) Retracts completely
    d) Remains the same
32. What part of the bull's body leaves the ground first when he mounts the cow?
    a) The head
    b) The tail
    c) The shoulder and forelegs
    d) The hind legs
33. How long does the copulatory mounting last in buffaloes?
    a) About an hour
    b) Several hours
    c) A few minutes
    d) Some tens of seconds
34. What happens specifically with the bull's abdominal muscles during mounting?
    a) The bull stands completely still.
    b) The bull relaxes its pelvic muscles.
    c) The external genitalia move backward
    d) The rectus abdominis muscles contract suddenly.
35. What happens after a bull ejaculates?
    a) The bull dismounts slowly
    b) The bull stays in place
    c) The bull falls asleep immediately.
    d) The bull runs away quickly.
36. Where is the semen ejaculated during the bull's ejaculatory thrust?
    a) Next to the prepuce.
    b) Outside of the body.
    c) Near the os-cervix.
    d) Inside the stomach.
37. What is the 'refractory period'?
    a) A period for physical rest after exercise
    b) A time of increased feeding after copulation
    c) A time when animals migrate
    d) A time of no sexual activity right after mating.
38. Who shows a refractory period after mating?
    a) Fish
    b) Birds
    c) Buffalo bulls
    d) Dogs
39. How can males quickly return to mounting behavior?
    a) By mating with a new oestrous female.
    b) By resting in a shaded area
    c) By drinking a lot of water.
    d) By eating more food.

40. What happens after the male buffalo has dismounted?
    a) He starts grazing and ignores the female.
    b) He goes to rest and does not return for a while.
    c) He usually continues to tend the female and mounts her again.
    d) He leaves the female and searches for another mate.
41. Which factor does NOT influence the frequency of copulation in buffaloes?
    a) The ratio of males and females
    b) The time of day
    c) The available space
    d) The breed of the buffaloes
42. Which animal has been observed to copulate up to 80 times within 24 hours?
    a) Stallion
    b) Bull
    c) Boar
    d) Ram
43. What happens to the copulation frequency of a ram after a long sexual rest?
    a) Copulates up to 50 times on the first day
    b) Does not copulate after rest
    c) Always copulates less than 10 times
    d) Copulates only 10 times on day first day
44. Which animals reach exhaustion after fewer ejaculations compared to bulls and rams?
    a) All animals the same
    b) Only rams
    c) Only bulls
    d) Goat, stallion, and boar
45. Which of the following factors affect duration of estrus?
    a) Breed, diet, climate, and habitat
    b) Species, diet, exercise, and temperature
    c) Species, breed, climate, and management
    d) Species, climate, exercise, and behavior
46. The penile erection in bulls is under control of ?
    a) Parasympathetic system
    b) Sympathetic system
    c) Both a & b
    d) Endocrine system
47. The parasympathetic nerves supply a bull's external genitalia arise feom?
    a) Thoracic segments of the spinal cord
    b) Sacral segments of the spinal cord
    c) Cervical segments of the spinal cord
    d) Lumbar segments of the spinal cord
48. The sexual desire in bull is elicited by ?
    a) Temperature and pressure clues
    b) Taste and smell clues
    c) Auditory and smell clues
    d) Visual and tactile clues
49. Which type of bulls are more sluggish?
    a) Dairy bulls
    b) Duroc bulls
    c) Brahman bulls
    d) Yorkshire bulls

50. Why are Yorkshire boars easier to train for semen collections?
   a) They are more cooperative
   b) They are smaller in size
   c) They sleep more
   d) They eat less
51. What aspect of sexual behavior shows more differences among identical twin bulls?
   a) The colour of their fur
   b) The size of the bulls
   c) The sound they make
   d) The pattern of sexual behavior
52. What happens to the male's libido when new females become receptive in the herd?
   a) It stops completely
   b) It decreases
   c) It increases
   d) It stays the same
53. What effect does changing the teaser bull have under modern husbandry conditions?
   a) Decreases the sexual behavior of a sluggish male
   b) Stops sexual behavior completely.
   c) No effect on sexual behavior
   d) Increases the sexual behavior of a sluggish male
54. What can help in encouraging sexual activity in males with low libido?
   a) Adjusting their sleep schedule
   b) Offering different toys.
   c) Changing the place of semen collection
   d) Increasing their food intake.
55. What improves the sexual libido of a male in the presence of other males?
   a) Teasing a female
   b) Eating a lot of food
   c) Fighting with other males
   d) Ignoring a female
56. Who performs most of the copulations when several males compete for one receptive female?
   a) The female herself
   b) The smallest male
   c) The dominant male
   d) The weakest male
57. What happens when females are in excess?
   a) Dominant males become inferior
   b) Males stop competing
   c) Dominant males cannot control their inferiors
   d) Females stop reproducing
58. Who usually dominates yearling rams?
   a) Younger yearling rams
   b) Older yearling rams
   c) Female rams
   d) Adult rams
59. What affects the competition among males in addition to social hierarchy?
   a) The age of males
   b) The weather condition
   c) The number of females
   d) The size of the pasture

60. Introduction of respective male of during "seasonal anestrus" in sheep and goats results in ?
   a) More wool production by sheep and goats
   b) Sheep and goats stop eating
   c) The Synchronized estrous cycles
   d) Sheep and goats start milking

61. How long after male introduction do sheep show the peak of estrus?
   a) 10 to 12 days b) 5 to 6 days
   c) 17 to 18 days d) 20 to 21 days

62. Which behavior is exhibited by male goats during the breeding season?
   a) Building nests b) Gathering food
   c) Self-urination d) Digging holes

63. What effect does the introduction of a boar have on isolated gilts?
   a) It makes them produce milk earlier
   b) Hasten onset of puberty
   c) It slows down their growth
   d) It causes them to eat more.

64. What is a common cause of inability to mount in older buffalo bulls?
   a) Lack of food
   b) Locomotor dysfunction or musculo-skeletal diseases
   c) Too much sunlight
   d) Too much exercise

65. What might help a bull regain interest if it refuses to mount?
   a) Changing the sexual stimulus to a new steer or bull
   b) Reducing its food intake
   c) Taking it for a walk
   d) Providing more water

66. What is a possible reason for a bull's penis being unable to enter the vagina?
   a) Haematoma of the penis b) Normal blood flow
   c) Healthy libido d) Frequent urination

67. What can cause the penis of a bull to be too flaccid to achieve intromission?
   a) Abnormal venous drainage b) Young age
   c) Good health d) Excessive exercise

68. What happens to a 'buller' in a feedlot herd?
   a) It becomes the leader of the herd
   d) It separates itself from the herd
   c) It attacks other animals
   d) It may be ridden to exhaustion or death

69. What can cause males in sex-aggregated groups to change their sexual behavior?
    a) Changing their diet.
    b) Being placed with females.
    c) Moving to a different location.
    d) Increasing their exercise

70. What is a characteristic of hyper-sexuality in males?
    a) Frequent copulation.
    b) No sexual desire.
    c) Lack of interest in females.
    d) Failure to ejaculate.

71. What is auto-erotic behaviour also known as in males?
    a) High protein ration
    b) Arched back movement
    c) Pelvic thrusting
    d) Masturbation

72. When do bulls most commonly masturbate?
    a) During times of inactivity
    b) During sleep
    c) During exercise
    d) During feeding

73. What is 'silent heat' in buffaloes?
    a) The failure to show signs of oestrus when ovulation is near
    b) The phase when buffaloes lose weight
    c) The time when buffaloes sleep more
    d) The period when buffaloes do not eat

74. Which condition can lead to reduced or no visible signs of heat in buffaloes during summer?
    a) Regular oestrus
    b) Submissive behaviour
    c) Active heat
    d) Silent heat

75. What can cause the cessation of oestrus behaviour in buffaloes?
    a) Heavy rain or snowfalls
    b) High food consumption
    c) Playing with other animals
    d) Excessive rest

76. Which of the following methods involves animals wearing equipment to assist in detecting cows in oestrus?
    a) Painting the tail and noting when the paint is scruffed off
    b) Training dogs to sniff out cows
    c) Using teaser or vasectomized bulls with a marking harness
    d) Measuring progesterone levels in milk

77. What is one of the methods used to automatically detect changes related to oestrus in cows?
    a) Training dogs to sniff out cows in oestrus
    b) Painting the tail and rump each day
    c) Changes in the physical activity as walking distance
    d) Using teaser bulls without any equipment

78. What is another name for nymphomania in cattle?
    a) Follicular Disease
    b) Milk Fever
    c) Bulling
    d) Cystic Ovary

79. What typically causes nymphomania in female cows?
    a) Lack of calcium
    b) Low water intake
    c) Ovarian cysts
    d) High protein diet
80. The behaviour of nymphomaniac cow is characterized by ?
    a) They stand still and are quiet
    b) They act like bulls and mount other cows
    c) They eat less and avoid other cows
    d) They seek human attention
81. Which behavior is commonly seen in nymphomaniac cows?
    a) Aggressively pursuing pawing the ground and bellowing
    b) Eating more food
    c) Drinking more water
    d) Sleeping more than usual
82. What physical changes are characteristic of a chronically nymphomaniac cow?
    a) Musculinization of the head and neck
    b) Brightly coloured fur
    c) Shorter legs
    d) Enlarged hooves
83. What is an important factor for satisfactory reproductive performance in mammals after calving?
    a) Reduction in body weight
    b) Increase in food intake
    c) Decreased lactation
    d) Resumption of oestrus cyclicity
84. When is pre-service anoestrus observed?
    a) After lactation ends
    b) In the immediate postpartum period
    c) During insemination
    d) During pregnancy
85. What are some physiopathological factors of anoestrus mentioned in the text?
    a) Cold season and hot season
    b) Lactation and infections
    c) Adequate oestrus detection
    d) Management practices only
86. Oestrus behaviour
    a) More pronounced in the cold season
    b) Same in all seasons
    c) More pronounced in the hot season
    d) Less pronounced in the cold season
87. Cause of anoestrus
    a) Maintenance of the corpus luteum
    b) Reduction in food intake
    c) Stress from calving
    d) Increased lactation
88. What is the main function of courtship behaviour?
    a) To show aggression
    b) To build a nest
    c) To find food
    d) To ensure individuals are of the same species

89. What does courtship behaviour informs a potential mate?
    a) That the intention is playing
    b) That the intention is establishing territory
    c) That the intention is finding food
    d) That the intention is breeding
90. How can the low copulatory behaviour of males be improved?
    a) By using smaller males
    b) By giving more food
    c) By changing the season
    d) By preventing males from slipping while mounting
91. What might frequent mounting events by a male stimulate in a female?
    a) Receptivity to mating
    b) Aggressiveness
    c) Hunger
    d) Sleepiness
92. What are nonejaculatory intromissions considered to be?
    a) Randomized actions in the wild
    b) Evolved signals in the tactile modality
    c) Signals in the visual modality
    d) Dangerous behaviors for organisms
93. Which analysis traditions can improve understanding of courtship behavior?
    a) Visual and audio
    b) Historical and cultural
    c) Classical ethological and sociobiological
    d) Mathematical and statistical
94. What do nonejaculatory intromissions in courtship help to do?
    a) Speed up, slow down, reverse, and pause
    b) Attract, repel, amplify, and dampen
    c) Synchronize, persuade, orient, and isolate
    d) Confuse, disguise, distract, and hide
95. Why is courtship communication considered within the context of copulatory behavior?
    a) To make it harder to understand
    b) To decide mating rituals
    c) To analyze patterns effectively
    d) To complicate the study
96. What influences the development of courtship behaviours and preferences in certain species?
    a) Social learning
    b) Genetic mutations
    c) Environmental changes
    d) Population size
97. How can behaviours that are transmitted socially spread through populations?
    a) Not at all
    b) Very quickly
    c) Only if they are genetic
    d) Quite slowly

98. What is the primary reason for the seasonal variations in sexual behavior of sheep, goats, and horses?
   a) Changes in nutrition
   b) Temperature fluctuations
   c) Seasonal changes in daylight
   d) Seasonality of hypothalamic/pituitary function

99. Which season is associated with the full expression of estrous behaviour in ovariectomized female goats when given an injection of 30 µg of estradiol?
   a) Fall b) Spring
   c) Summer d) Winter

100. What does the replicated experiment in environmentally controlled rooms suggest about sexual behavior?
   a) Importance of photoperiod b) Impact of animal's age
   c) Critical role of temperature d) Significance of nutrition

101. How are ovariectomized ewes, does, and sows affected by exogenous hormones according to the text?
   a) Genetically b) Permanently
   c) Randomly d) Seasonally

102. What environmental factor reduces the intensity of sexual behavior?
   a) High nutrition levels b) Hot climates
   c) Cold climates d) Low daylight

Answer Key

1	b	2	b	3	d	4	a	5	a	6	b	7	d
8	c	9	b	10	d	11	b	12	a	13	b	14	b
15	c	16	d	17	a	18	a	19	c	20	c	21	a
22	a	23	a	24	d	25	c	26	d	27	a	28	d
29	b	30	d	31	b	32	c	33	d	34	d	35	a
36	c	37	d	38	c	39	a	40	c	41	b	42	b
43	a	44	d	45	c	46	a	47	b	48	d	49	c
50	a	51	d	52	c	53	d	54	c	55	a	56	c
57	c	58	d	59	d	60	c	61	c	62	c	63	b
64	b	65	a	66	a	67	a	68	d	69	b	70	a
71	d	72	a	73	a	74	d	75	a	76	c	77	c
78	c	79	c	80	b	81	a	82	a	83	d	84	b
85	b	86	a	87	a	88	d	89	d	90	d	91	a
92	b	93	c	94	c	95	c	96	a	97	b	98	d
99	a	100	a	101	d	102	b						

5

Habituation Sensitization and Conditioning

S.S.R. Kona[1], M.P.S. Tomar[1], S.K.I. Vasantha[1] and Kush Shrivastava[2]

[1]Sri Venkateswara Veterinary University, Tirupati, Andhra Pradesh

[2]Animal Biotechnology Centre, Nanaji Deshmukh Veterinary Science University Jabalpur, Madhya Pradesh

Introduction

A significant aspect of an animal's existence is their adaptability to changing circumstances and their willingness to adapt their behaviour. An animal becomes more intelligent the more it learns. Associative and non-associative learning are the two main categories into which learning can be divided. Whereas associative learning involves classical conditioning, non-associative learning involves sensitization and habituation. When a stimulus occurs frequently, an individual develops a gradual familiarity with it. This is known as habituation. Sensitization, on the other hand, is the increased response to the same stimulus that may or may not be related to other variables. In order to get the desired response, training is required for the behavioural responses to two independent stimuli that are kept associated during the conditioning process. In general, non-associative learning stems from an animal's perception of its environment or circumstances, whereas conditioning is based on training-based learning.

MCQ's

1. Animals habituate quickly to common environmental sounds and no longer react to them is called as
   - a) Habituation
   - b) Dishabituation
   - c) Conditioning
   - d) All the above
2. Increase in frequency or probability of a behavioral response to a given stimulus is called as
   - a) Desensitization
   - b) Conditioning
   - c) Sensitization
   - d) Dishabituation
3. Instrumental conditioning was first investigated by
   - a) B.F. Skinner
   - b) P. Pavlov
   - c) Both a and b
   - d) None of the above

4. The form of learning in which behaviour is learned, maintained changed through its consequences is
   a) Classical conditioning b) Insight Learning
   c) Habituation d) Instrumental conditioning
5. Any stimulus or event, which increases the probability of the occurrence of a (desired) response is defined as
   a) Reinforcer b) Operants
   c) Both a and b d) None of the above
6. The ability to respond correctly at the first time when an animal encounters a certain situation is known as
   a) Habituation b) Dishabituation
   c) Conditioning d) Insight Learning
7. The model of learning which could not be readily explained by conditioning is demonstrated by
   a) Kohler b) B.F. Skinner
   c) P. Pavlov d) All the above
8. Insight Learning was demonstrated by
   a) P. Pavlov b) B.F. Skinner
   c) Kohler d) None of the above
9. The form of learning that occurs without any obvious reinforcement of the behavior or associations that are learned
   a) Latent learning b) Insight Learning
   c) Imprinting d) Instrumental conditioning
10. Who made an early contribution to the concept of latent learning
   a) Kohler b) B.F. Skinner
   c) P. Pavlov d) Tolman
11. The kind of phase-sensitive learning (learning occurring at a particular age or a particular life stage) that is rapid and apparently independent of the consequences of behavior is called
   a) Imprinting b) Dishabituation
   c) Conditioning d) Insight Learning
12. Young Chicks following their mother belongs to which type of imprinting
   a) Sexual imprinting b) Filial imprinting
   c) Habituation d) All the above
13. The process by which a young animal learns the characteristics of a desirable mate is called as
   a) Habituation b) Filial imprinting
   c) Sexual imprinting d) All the above

14. The individual becomes gradually familiar with a stimulus when it comes repeatedly is known as
    a) Habituation b) Dishabituation
    c) Conditioning d) Insight Learning
15. The increased response for the same stimulus which may or may not be associated to other factors is known as
    a) Habituation b) Sensitization
    c) Conditioning d) Classical conditioning
16. Classical conditioning belongs to which type of learning
    a) Non-associative learning b) Associative learning
    c) Both a and b d) None of the above
17. The non-associative learning includes
    a) Habituation b) Sensitization
    c) Both a and b d) None of the above
18. In which species Ivan P. Pavlov conducted experiments for Classical conditioning
    a) Rabbit b) Dog
    c) Guineapig d) Rat
19. The early form of social learning seen in some species like chickens, ducks, geese and turkeys is
    a) Imprinting b) Dishabituation
    c) Conditioning d) Insight Learning
20. B.F. Skinner called the organisms used in instrumental conditioning study as
    a) Imprinters b) Operants
    c) Both a and b d) None of the above
21. In which species Skinner conducted his studies of instrumental conditioning
    a) Rats b) Pigeons
    c) Both a and b d) None of the above
22. In which species Kohler performed a series of experiments in order to explain insight learning
    a) Chimpanzees b) Dogs
    c) Chicks d) All the above
23. In which species Tolman conducted his experiments to explain latent learning
    a) Chimpanzees b) Dogs
    c) Chicks d) Rats
24. The process by which the solution to a problem suddenly becomes clear is called
    a) Imprinting b) Dishabituation
    c) Conditioning d) Insight Learning

25. Pavlov experiments on dog, salivation started to occur in the presence of the sound of the bell without food, here saliva secretion is
    a) Unconditioned Stimulus (US)
    b) Unconditioned Response (UR)
    c) Conditioned Stimulus (CS)
    d) Conditioned Response (CR)
26. The ability to recognize surroundings and memorize a route is which type of learning
    a) Latent learning
    b) Insight Learning
    c) Imprinting
    d) Spatial learning
27. The type of learning usually tested in the laboratory as maze learning is
    a) Classical conditioning
    b) Insight Learning
    c) Spatial learning
    d) Instrumental conditioning
28. The type of learning involves an unconditioned stimulus that elicits a response is known as
    a) Classical conditioning
    b) Insight Learning
    c) Spatial learning
    d) Instrumental conditioning
29. The type of conditioning occurs when the animal does something to receive a reward is known as
    a) Classical conditioning
    b) Operant conditioning
    c) Spatial learning
    d) Instrumental conditioning
30. The type of learning occurs most frequently in response to nausea and is associated with taste or odour is called as
    a) Classical conditioning
    b) Operant conditioning
    c) Conditioned taste aversion
    d) Instrumental conditioning
31. The behavioural responses for two independent stimuli kept associated and it needs training to get the desired response is known as
    a) Desensitization
    b) Conditioning
    c) Sensitization
    d) Dishabituation
32. Learning based on animals' own perception about their surrounding or situation is known as
    a) Non-associative learning
    b) Associative learning
    c) Spatial learning
    d) None of the above
33. Habituation becomes progressively faster with repeated series of training sessions, this phenomenon of habituation and spontaneous recovery is called as
    a) Potentiation of habituation
    b) Instrumental conditioning
    c) Dishabituation
    d) None of the above
34. A second, novel stimulus is given, and the differences in the responses to the novel stimulus and the habituated stimulus are compared, the test used in order to assess stimulus specificity is
    a) Stimulus generalisation test
    b) Operant conditioning
    c) Conditioned taste aversion
    d) Instrumental conditioning

35. The squirrels' peaceful coexistence in the wild or in a park with the people who frequent or live nearby is an example of_______________
    a) Habituation b) Dishabituation
    c) Conditioning d) All the above
36. A turtle's head retracts when it is touched; nevertheless, it cannot conceal or retract its head if it is repeatedly touched is an example of________
    a) Habituation b) Dishabituation
    c) Conditioning d) None of the above
37. Sensitization to the sound of honey bees will protect elephants from sting bites is an example of_______________
    a) Habituation b) Sensitization
    c) Conditioning d) All the above
38. Dogs that are frequently exposed to fireworks and thunderstorms develop a fear of other unexpected noises is an example of
    a) Habituation b) Sensitization
    c) Conditioning d) All of the above
39. Russian scientist Ivan Pavlov experiments on dogs is an example of
    a) Classical conditioning b) Operant conditioning
    c) Conditioned taste aversion d) Instrumental conditioning
40. Ducks' habit of interacting with people all the time and feeding them without any threat is an example of
    a) Habituation b) Sensitization
    c) Conditioning d) None of the above

Answer Key

1	b	2	c	3	a	4	d	5	a	6	d	7	a
8	c	9	a	10	d	11	a	12	b	13	c	14	a
15	b	16	b	17	c	18	b	19	a	20	b	21	c
22	a	23	d	24	c	25	d	26	d	27	c	28	a
29	b	30	c	31	b	32	a	33	a	34	a	35	a
36	a	37	b	38	b	39	a	40	a				

6

Innate and Adaptive Behavior

Preeti Lakhani[1], Amrapali Bhimte[2] and Gaurav Dixit[1]

[1]*Department of Veterinary Physiology and Biochemistry, Lala Lajpat Rai University of Veterinary and Animal Sciences, Hisar, Harayana*

[2]*Department of Veterinary Physiology and Biochemistry, Nanaji Deshmukh Veterinary Sciences University, Jabalpur, Madhya Pradesh*

Introduction

Innate and adaptive behaviors are fundamental aspects of the behavioral repertoire exhibited by organisms across the biological spectrum. This abstract provides an overview of the key characteristics, mechanisms, and evolutionary significance of these two distinct forms of behavior.Innate behavior refers to genetically programmed actions or responses that are typically present from birth or shortly after. These behaviors are often instinctual and do not require prior learning or experience. They are crucial for the survival and reproduction of an organism, encompassing actions such as feeding, mating, and predator avoidance. Innate behaviors are deeply rooted in an organism's biology and are thought to have evolved as a result of natural selection to optimize an individual's chances of survival and reproductive success. On the other hand, adaptive behavior encompasses actions that are learned or modified through experience and environmental interactions. Adaptive behaviors are highly flexible and can vary among individuals of the same species. These behaviors allow organisms to adjust to changing environmental conditions, exploit new resources, and navigate social interactions. Learning and memory play a central role in the development of adaptive behaviors, enabling organisms to refine their responses over time.This abstract also highlights the interplay between innate and adaptive behavior in many organisms. While innate behaviors provide a foundational framework for survival, adaptive behaviors allow individuals to fine-tune their responses and maximize their fitness in dynamic environments. The relationship between these two types of behaviors is complex and varies depending on the species and its ecological niche.Understanding the mechanisms and interactions between innate and adaptive behavior is crucial for researchers in fields such as ethology, psychology, and ecology. By investigating the intricate interplay of these behaviors, scientists gain insight into the evolutionary forces shaping the behavioral diversity observed in the natural world. This knowledge has broad implications for fields ranging from wildlife conservation to human psychology and may inform strategies for improving the well-being and adaptability of species, including our own.

MCQ's

1. Innate behavior is:
   a) Learned through experience
   b) Determined by genetics
   c) Acquired through social interactions
   d) Developed through trial and error
2. Which of the following is an example of innate behavior in animals?
   a) A dog learning to sit on command
   b) A bird building a nest
   c) A spider spinning a web
   d) A cat chasing a laser pointer
3. Innate behavior is also known as:
   a) Reflex behavior
   b) Conditioned behavior
   c) Observational behavior
   d) Voluntary behavior
4. Which of the following is NOT an example of innate behavior in humans?
   a) Sucking reflex in newborns
   b) Crying when experiencing pain
   c) Learning to ride a bicycle
   d) Smiling in response to a happy face
5. Imprinting is an example of:
   a) Innate behavior
   b) Learned behavior
   c) Social behavior
   d) Habituation
6. Courtship displays in animals are primarily driven by:
   a) Innate behavior
   b) Learned behavior
   c) Cultural influences
   d) Environmental factors
7. Which of the following is an example of a fixed action pattern?
   a) A bird building a nest
   b) A dog learning to fetch a ball
   c) A spider spinning a web
   d) A squirrel burying nuts
8. Innate behavior is:
   a) Universal across all species
   b) Present only in humans
   c) Present only in animals
   d) Variable across different species
9. The ability of a newborn baby to root for a nipple is an example of:
   a) Innate behavior
   b) Learned behavior
   c) Social behavior
   d) Habituation
10. Innate behavior is:
    a) Rigid and unchangeable
    b) Flexible and adaptable
    c) Only present in mammals
    d) Learned through trial and error
11. Innate behavior is:
    a) Learned through experience
    b) Genetically programmed
    c) Acquired from peers
    d) Developed through trial and error

12. Which of the following statements is true about innate behavior?
    a) It is always flexible and can be modified.
    b) It is only exhibited by higher organisms.
    c) It requires a complex neural system.
    d) It is instinctive and does not require prior experience.
13. Which of the following is an example of innate behavior in animals?
    a) A dog performing tricks after being trained by its owner.
    b) A bird building a nest based on observation of other birds.
    c) A spider weaving a web without any prior experience.
    d) A cat learning to use a litter box through trial and error.
14. Which of the following is an example of a fixed action pattern (FAP)?
    a) A bird learning to mimic human speech.
    b) A spider constructing a web in response to vibrations.
    c) A dog being trained to fetch a ball.
    d) A monkey solving a puzzle to receive a reward.
15. Imprinting is a type of innate behavior observed in:
    a) Humans b) Insects
    c) Birds d) Reptiles
16. Migration is an example of which type of innate behavior?
    a) Taxis b) Reflexes
    c) Hibernation d) Fixed action pattern
17. Which of the following is an example of innate behavior in humans?
    a) Speaking a language
    b) Playing a musical instrument
    c) Sucking reflex in infants
    d) Solving complex mathematical problems
18. The startle reflex, where a person reacts to a sudden loud noise, is an example of:
    a) Innate behavior b) Learned behavior
    c) Habituation d) Operant conditioning
19. Phototaxis is an innate behavior observed in:
    a) Plants b) Bacteria
    c) Birds d) Mammals
20. Which of the following animals exhibits a mating ritual as an innate behavior?
    a) Honeybees b) Cheetahs
    c) Sharks d) Dolphins
21. The instinctive migration of monarch butterflies is an example of:
    a) Fixed action patterns b) Hibernation
    c) Taxis d) Reflexes

22. Which of the following is a characteristic of adaptive behavior?
    a) It is genetically programmed and fixed.
    b) It is rigid and inflexible.
    c) It increases an organism's chances of survival and reproduction.
    d) It is solely learned through experience.
23. Adaptive behavior is shaped by:
    a) Genetic mutations.
    b) Environmental factors.
    c) Cultural influences.
    d) Random chance events.
24. Which of the following is an example of adaptive behavior in animals?
    a) A dog performing tricks for entertainment.
    b) A bird building a nest to attract a mate.
    c) A cat hunting and catching prey.
    d) A monkey solving a puzzle for a reward.
25. What is the primary driver of adaptive behavior?
    a) Genetic predisposition
    b) Environmental stimuli
    c) Social influences
    d) Behavioral conditioning
26. Camouflage is an example of adaptive behavior primarily used for:
    a) Attracting a mate
    b) Warning potential predators
    c) Finding food sources
    d) Evading predators
27. Which of the following is an example of a learned adaptive behavior?
    a) A sea turtle returning to its birthplace to lay eggs.
    b) A squirrel burying nuts for winter storage.
    c) A bee performing a waggle dance to communicate food location.
    d) A salmon swimming upstream to spawn.
28. Adaptive behavior can be influenced by:
    a) Natural selection
    b) Cultural practices
    c) Individual choice
    d) Random chance
29. Migration is an example of adaptive behavior primarily driven by:
    a) Seasonal changes
    b) Social hierarchies
    c) Genetic programming
    d) Availability of resources
30. Which of the following is an example of adaptive behavior in humans?
    a) Sweating to regulate body temperature
    b) Playing video games for entertainment
    c) Using tools to build shelter
    d) Listening to music for relaxation
31. The ability of a chameleon to change its skin color to match its surroundings is an example of:
    a) Mimicry
    b) Reflexes
    c) Habituation
    d) Adaptive behavior

32. Habituation is best described as:
    a) A learned response to a new stimulus.
    b) An innate behavior observed in animals.
    c) The process of becoming more sensitive to a stimulus over time.
    d) The decrease in response to a repeated or prolonged stimulus.
33. Which of the following is an example of habituation?
    a) A dog wagging its tail when it sees its owner.
    b) A person getting scared by a loud noise.
    c) A bird building a nest.
    d) A person no longer noticing the sound of traffic outside their window.
34. Habituation is most closely associated with which type of learning?
    a) Classical conditioning
    b) Operant conditioning
    c) Observational learning
    d) Trial and error learning
35. The habituation process involves:
    a) Increasing the response to a repeated stimulus.
    b) Ignoring the stimulus completely.
    c) Decreasing the response to a repeated stimulus.
    d) Reacting differently to each presentation of the stimulus.
36. Habituation is an adaptive behavior because:
    a) It helps organisms learn new behaviors.
    b) It allows organisms to respond to any stimulus in their environment.
    c) It conserves energy by reducing unnecessary responses to familiar stimuli.
    d) It helps organisms establish social connections with others.
37. Which of the following factors can influence habituation?
    a) Age of the organism
    b) Intensity of the stimulus
    c) Frequency of stimulus presentation
    d) All of the above
38. Spontaneous recovery refers to:
    a) The sudden reappearance of a response after a period of non-exposure to the stimulus.
    b) The gradual decrease in response to a stimulus over time.
    c) The transfer of a learned response to a similar stimulus.
    d) The process of generalizing a response to different situations.
39. Habituation can occur in:
    a) Humans only
    b) Animals only
    c) Both humans and animals
    d) Neither humans nor animals
40. Which of the following is an example of habituation in everyday life?
    a) Becoming accustomed to the smell of a new perfume.
    b) Learning to play a musical instrument.
    c) Solving a crossword puzzle.
    d) Observing a friend perform a dance routine.

41. Dishabituation occurs when:
    a) A new stimulus is introduced and the response increases again.
    b) The response to a repeated stimulus remains constant.
    c) The response to a stimulus decreases over time.
    d) The response to a stimulus becomes more intense with repetition.

42. Innate behaviors are:
    a) Genetically programmed and do not require prior experience
    b) Acquired through experience and observation
    c) Only observed in humans, not in animals
    d) Developed through higher-order cognitive processes

43. An organism's response to a specific stimulus without prior experience is known as:
    a) Classical conditioning
    b) Innate behavior
    c) Observational learning
    d) Cognitive learning

44. Observing and imitating the actions of others is a characteristic of:
    a) Classical conditioning
    b) Innate behavior
    c) Observational learning
    d) Cognitive learning

45. Which of the following is NOT an example of an innate behavior?
    a) A spider spinning a web
    b) A newborn baby grasping onto a finger
    c) A human learning to play a musical instrument
    d) A snake shedding its skin

46. Adaptive behavior refers to behaviors that:
    a) Are genetically programmed and instinctive
    b) Are learned through experience and observation
    c) Are disadvantageous and harmful to an organism
    d) Help an organism adjust to its environment and promote survival

47. Which of the following is an example of adaptive behavior?
    a) A deer running away from a predator
    b) A cat grooming itself
    c) A bird singing a mating call
    d) A fish swimming in a school

48. Adaptive behaviors are essential for an organism's:
    a) Genetic development
    b) Survival and reproduction
    c) Ability to solve complex puzzles
    d) Capacity for observational learning

49. The primary purpose of adaptive behavior is to:
    a) Reinforce innate behaviors
    b) Support the development of cognitive skills
    c) Facilitate social interactions
    d) Enhance an organism's chances of survival and reproduction

50. Which of the following is an example of adaptive behavior in a social context?
   a) A lion hunting for prey
   b) A monkey grooming another monkey to strengthen social bonds
   c) A butterfly going through metamorphosis
   d) A bird building a nest

51. Adaptive behaviors are typically:
   a) Rigid and unchangeable
   b) Genetically determined and instinctive
   c) Highly variable and unpredictable
   d) Flexible and can be modified based on environmental demands

52. The ability of an organism to adjust its behavior in response to changes in its environment is an example of:
   a) Innate behavior
   b) Observational learning
   c) Adaptive behavior
   d) Classical conditioning

53. Adaptive behaviors can be influenced by:
   a) Genetic factors only
   b) Environmental factors only
   c) Both genetic and environmental factors
   d) Cognitive abilities

54. Which of the following is an example of adaptive behavior in a human context?
   a) A baby crying for food
   b) A person learning a new language
   c) A dog fetching a ball
   d) A plant growing towards sunlight

55. Adaptive behaviors can be influenced by:
   a) Genetic factors only
   b) Environmental factors only
   c) Both genetic and environmental factors
   d) Cognitive abilities

56. Which of the following types of genes are primarily associated with innate behaviors?
   a) Regulatory genes
   b) Learning genes
   c) Adaptive genes
   d) Instinct genes

57. Adaptive behaviors are influenced by genes that:
   a) Are fixed and unchangeable
   b) Encode specific learning experiences
   c) Provide a genetic basis for flexible responses
   d) Control innate reflexes

58. The genes responsible for encoding instinctive behaviors are often involved in the development of:
   a) Learning abilities
   b) Neural plasticity
   c) Instinctive responses
   d) Cognitive function

59. Which type of genes play a significant role in shaping the cognitive processes involved in adaptive behavior?
   a) Regulatory genes
   b) Instinct genes
   c) Learning genes
   d) Developmental genes

60. The genetic basis of adaptive behaviors allows for:
  a) Innate reflexes
  b) Rigid and unchangeable responses
  c) Adaptation to changing environments
  d) Instinctive behaviors only

61. In the context of adaptive behaviors, what role do regulatory genes play?
  a) Encoding instinctive responses
  b) Modulating gene expression based on environmental cues
  c) Controlling learning abilities
  d) Influencing cognitive functions

62. Which of the following statements about genes and adaptive behaviors is correct?
  a) Genes only influence innate behaviors, not adaptive ones.
  b) Adaptive behaviors are solely shaped by learning experiences, not genes.
  c) The interplay between genes and the environment contributes to adaptive behaviors.
  d) Genes play a minor role in adaptive behaviors compared to instincts.

63. Which type of hormones are involved in the stress response, a crucial aspect of adaptive behavior?
  a) Thyroid hormones b) Growth hormones
  c) Adrenal hormones d) Gonadal hormones

64. Adaptive behaviors related to reproduction are influenced by hormones released by the:
  a) Pituitary gland b) Thyroid gland
  c) Adrenal glands d) Gonads (testes or ovaries)

65. The endocrine system communicates with the brain through:
  a) Hormonal receptors on neurons
  b) Electrical signals sent via nerves
  c) Direct interaction with neurotransmitters
  d) The blood-brain barrier

66. Hormones released by the endocrine system can directly influence which of the following processes involved in adaptive behavior?
  a) Learning and memory
  b) Muscular strength and endurance
  c) Problem-solving and decision-making
  d) Sensory perception

67. In the context of innate behavior, hormonal fluctuations can lead to:
  a) Increased flexibility and adaptability
  b) Changes in behavior based on learning experiences
  c) Fixed and unalterable responses
  d) A lack of genetic influence

68. The hypothalamic-pituitary-adrenal (HPA) axis is involved in regulating hormonal responses to:
    a) Stress
    b) Hunger
    c) Social interactions
    d) Reproductive behaviors
69. The area of the brain associated with language comprehension and production is called:
    a) Broca's area
    b) Wernicke's area
    c) Heschl's gyrus
    d) Superior colliculus
70. The brain's ability to change and adapt in response to experiences is known as:
    a) Neurotransmission
    b) Neural plasticity
    c) Neurogenesis
    d) Synaptic pruning
71. Which of the following hormones is commonly associated with the fight-or-flight response and can influence both innate and adaptive behaviors?
    a) Insulin
    b) Estrogen
    c) Cortisol
    d) Thyroxine
72. During social interactions, the hormone oxytocin is known to:
    a) Increase aggressive behavior
    b) Inhibit bonding and affiliative behaviors
    c) Promote trust and bonding
    d) Suppress reproductive behaviors
73. Testosterone, a hormone primarily associated with male development, has been linked to:
    a) Reduced risk-taking behavior
    b) Increased nurturing behavior in females
    c) Decreased territorial aggression in males
    d) Enhanced spatial memory in both sexes
74. Serotonin, a neurotransmitter that also has hormonal effects, is involved in regulating:
    a) Sleep-wake cycles
    b) Bone growth
    c) Blood glucose levels
    d) Muscle contraction
75. Prolactin, a hormone traditionally associated with lactation, can also influence behavior by:
    a) Enhancing appetite and food intake
    b) Inhibiting maternal behaviors
    c) Promoting paternal care in some species
    d) Reducing social interactions
76. The "fight or flight" response is primarily mediated by the release of which hormone?
    a) Estrogen
    b) Progesterone
    c) Adrenaline (epinephrine)
    d) Melatonin

77. Which hormone plays a crucial role in regulating the sleep-wake cycle and can affect mood and cognitive functions?

a) Insulin
b) Thyroxine
c) Melatonin
d) Testosterone

78. The hormone ghrelin is known to influence:

a) Bone growth
b) Hunger and appetite
c) Blood clotting
d) Stress response

79. Cortisol, often referred to as the "stress hormone," can impact behavior by:

a) Inducing relaxation and calmness
b) Enhancing memory and cognitive functions
c) Promoting immune system suppression
d) Increasing alertness and preparing for challenges

80. In the context of maternal behavior, which hormone is linked to the development of nurturing behaviors and the formation of the mother-infant bond?

a) Testosterone
b) Oxytocin
c) Insulin
d) Progesterone

81. The term "phenotypic plasticity" refers to the ability of an organism to:

a) Pass on learned behaviors to its offspring
b) Adapt its behavior based on genetic predispositions
c) Modify its behavior in response to environmental cues
d) Exhibit consistent behaviors regardless of the environment

82. An example of an adaptive behavior influenced by environmental factors is:

a) Instinctual mating calls
b) Reflexive responses to sensory stimuli
c) Migration patterns in birds
d) Inherited fear of predators

83. The concept of "critical periods" in development suggests that certain behaviors are most effectively learned:

a) During adulthood
b) At any time throughout an organism's life
c) Only during infancy or specific developmental stages
d) Exclusively through genetic inheritance

84. The process of habituation involves:

a) Enhancing a natural behavior through repeated practice
b) Decreasing responsiveness to repeated or irrelevant stimuli
c) Replacing innate behaviors with learned behaviors
d) Establishing new behaviors through social interactions

85. Imprinting is a phenomenon seen in many animals where young animals form strong attachments to:
    a) Any moving object they encounter
    b) Their own reflection in a mirror
    c) Animals of their own species during a sensitive period
    d) The first human they see after birth
86. Social learning, a type of adaptive behavior, involves acquiring new behaviors by:
    a) Genetic inheritance
    b) Observing and imitating others
    c) Instinctual responses to environmental cues
    d) Spontaneous trial-and-error experimentation
87. Which of the following best exemplifies a learned behavior influenced by environmental factors?
    a) A spider spinning a web
    b) A cat grooming itself
    c) A dog salivating at the sound of a bell
    d) A chimpanzee using tools to extract termites from a mound
88. An animal's ability to navigate its environment using landmarks is an example of:
    a) A fixed action pattern
    b) Genetic determinism
    c) Spatial learning
    d) Epigenetic inheritance
89. In the context of humans, an example of an innate behavior that can be influenced by the environment is:
    a) Reflexive blinking in response to bright light
    b) Basic motor skills like crawling
    c) The development of complex language abilities
    d) The formation of personal preferences and tastes
90. Adaptive behaviors are those that an organism:
    a) Inherits genetically and can't change
    b) Develops through hormonal changes
    c) Acquires through learning and interaction with the environment
    d) Exhibits only during certain developmental stages
91. The nervous system plays a central role in adaptive behavior by:
    a) Determining genetic traits
    b) Influencing innate behaviors exclusively
    c) Processing sensory information and coordinating responses
    d) Regulating only hormonal functions
92. Neurons are the basic building blocks of the nervous system and are responsible for:
    a) Producing hormones
    b) Transmitting electrical signals
    c) Synthesizing enzymes
    d) Regulating metabolic processes

93. The junction between two neurons where information is transmitted is called a:
   a) Synaptic cleft
   b) Dendritic terminal
   c) Nodal point
   d) Myelin sheath
94. Which part of the neuron receives signals from other neurons or sensory receptors?
   a) Axon
   b) Cell body (soma)
   c) Synapse
   d) Dendrites
95. Neurotransmitters are chemicals that:
   a) Convert electrical signals into light
   b) Generate electric currents within neurons
   c) Transmit signals across synapses
   d) Regulate the heartbeat
96. The "fight or flight" response is triggered by the activation of the:
   a) Parasympathetic nervous system
   b) Somatic nervous system
   c) Sympathetic nervous system
   d) Central nervous system
97. The process by which neurons become more efficient at transmitting signals due to repeated use is known as:
   a) Synaptic pruning
   b) Neural plasticity
   c) Myelination
   d) Habituation
98. Which division of the nervous system is responsible for controlling involuntary functions such as heartbeat and digestion?
   a) Central nervous system
   b) Somatic nervous system
   c) Autonomic nervous system
   d) Peripheral nervous system
99. Plasticity in the nervous system refers to its ability to:
   a) Generate new neurons throughout life
   b) Change and reorganize in response to experience
   c) Store unlimited amounts of information
   d) Control innate behaviors without learning
100. What is the process by which an individual acquires new knowledge or skills through experience?
   a) Innate behavior
   b) Adaptation
   c) Learning
   d) Instinct
101. Which type of learning is characterized by associating a neutral stimulus with an unconditioned stimulus to produce a conditioned response?
   a) Operant conditioning
   b) Classical conditioning
   c) Observational learning
   d) Habituation
102. In operant conditioning, what is the consequence that strengthens a behavior and makes it more likely to be repeated?
   a) Neutral stimulus
   b) Unconditioned stimulus
   c) Reinforcement
   d) Punishment

103. Which type of learning occurs through observation and imitation of the behavior of others?
   a) Classical conditioning
   b) Operant conditioning
   c) Social learning
   d) Habituation

104. Habituation is a form of learning that involves:
   a) Associating a neutral stimulus with a conditioned stimulus.
   b) Reducing responsiveness to a repeated or irrelevant stimulus.
   c) Reinforcing a behavior through rewards.
   d) Associating a behavior with its consequences.

105. Which of the following is an example of positive reinforcement?
   a) A child loses a privilege for misbehaving.
   b) A dog is given a treat for performing a trick.
   c) A student is scolded for not completing their homework.
   d) A driver gets a speeding ticket for exceeding the speed limit.

106. What is a primary reinforcer?
   a) A stimulus that initially has no significance but becomes reinforcing through association.
   b) A reward that fulfills a biological need, such as food or water.
   c) A punishment for undesirable behavior.
   d) A conditioned stimulus in classical conditioning.

107. Which learning theory emphasizes the role of cognition, thoughts, and mental processes in shaping behavior?
   a) Classical conditioning
   b) Operant conditioning
   c) Social learning theory
   d) Cognitive theory

108. What is extinction in the context of operant conditioning?
   a) The sudden appearance of a conditioned response to a neutral stimulus.
   b) The weakening and eventual disappearance of a conditioned response.
   c) The involuntary reaction to a conditioned stimulus.
   d) The process of forming an association between two stimuli.

109. In classical conditioning, what is the term for a previously neutral stimulus that, after being paired with an unconditioned stimulus, triggers a conditioned response?
   a) Reinforcement
   b) Extinction
   c) Neutral stimulus
   d) Habituation Top of Form

110. What is territorial behavior in animals primarily associated with?
   a) Finding mates
   b) Obtaining food
   c) Avoiding predators
   d) Defending a defined area

111. Territorial behavior is often related to which of the following ecological principles?
   a) Predation
   b) Symbiosis
   c) Resource distribution
   d) Camouflage

112. Which of the following is a benefit of territorial behavior for animals?
   a) Increased competition with neighbors
   b) Reduced access to potential mates
   c) Greater access to essential resources
   d) Enhanced susceptibility to predation
113. In the context of animal territories, what is a "home range"?
   a) The specific area within the territory where the animal feeds.
   b) The area within the territory where mating takes place.
   c) The core area an animal defends most vigorously.
   d) The entire area an animal travels within its territory.
114. What is the primary purpose of territorial displays in animals?
   a) To mark boundaries with scent marks
   b) To intimidate potential intruders
   c) To attract potential mates
   d) To communicate with other species
115. Which of the following is an example of an animal using scent marking for territorial behavior?
   a) A lion defending its pride's hunting grounds
   b) A peacock displaying its colorful feathers
   c) A hummingbird building a nest
   d) A fish swimming in a school
116. Territorial behavior is most commonly observed in which of the following animal groups?
   a) Herbivores
   b) Insects
   c) Marine mammals
   d) Migratory birds
117. What is the primary purpose of vocalizations in territorial communication among birds?
   a) To locate food sources
   b) To attract a mate
   c) To deter intruders
   d) To establish dominance within the territory
118. Which of the following is a disadvantage of territorial behavior in animals?
   a) Enhanced access to resources
   b) Decreased reproductive opportunities
   c) Increased vulnerability to predation
   d) Reduced communication with neighboring individuals

119. In the context of territorial disputes, what is "natal philopatry"?
   a) The tendency of animals to return to their birthplace to establish territories.
   b) The use of chemical signals to mark boundaries.
   c) The establishment of a territory near a water source.
   d) The sharing of territories between two individuals.

120. What is insight behavior in animals primarily associated with?
   a) Instinctual actions
   b) Trial-and-error learning
   c) Inherited genetic traits
   d) Classical conditioning

121. Insight behavior is often characterized by:
   a) Pre-established and automatic responses
   b) Sudden and novel problem-solving
   c) Innate and fixed actions
   d) Conditional reflexes

122. Who is known for his research on insight learning in chimpanzees, particularly his studies with a chimp named Sultan?
   a) Ivan Pavlov
   b) B.F. Skinner
   c) Edward Thorndike
   d) Wolfgang Köhler

123. In insight learning, when an animal solves a problem without a series of gradual steps, it is often referred to as:
   a) Habituation
   b) Classical conditioning
   c) The "Aha!" moment
   d) Operant conditioning

124. Which of the following best describes the typical process of insight learning?
   a) Repeatedly performing the same action until successful
   b) Gradually refining a behavior through trial and error
   c) Instantly recognizing a solution to a problem
   d) Associating a conditioned stimulus with an unconditioned response

125. Insight learning is often associated with which of the following cognitive abilities in animals?
   a) Memory retention
   b) Logical reasoning
   c) Classical conditioning
   d) Instinctual behaviors

126. Which animal is known for its ability to demonstrate insight learning in various problem-solving tasks, including using tools?
   a) Dolphins
   b) Crows
   c) Bees
   d) Snakes

127. Insight learning is considered a higher form of learning because it involves:
   a) Reflexive actions
   b) Inherited behaviors
   c) The use of prior experiences to solve novel problems
   d) Repetitive trial-and-error approaches

128. Which term is often used to describe insight learning in the context of animal behavior?

a) Conditioning
b) Imitation
c) Cognition
d) Habituation

129. In Wolfgang Köhler's famous studies with chimpanzees, what was one of the tasks that demonstrated insight learning?

a) Associating a bell ring with food
b) Stacking crates to reach a banana
c) Pressing a lever for a reward
d) Dancing to a specific rhythm

130. What is social behavior in animals primarily related to?

a) Solitary living
b) Isolation from conspecifics
c) Interactions with other members of the same species
d) Predatory behavior

131. Which of the following is an example of social behavior in animals?

a) A solitary lion hunting for prey
b) A group of meerkats cooperating to watch for predators
c) A bird building a nest on its own
d) A solitary turtle laying eggs in a burrow

132. Social behavior in animals can involve various activities, including:

a) Territorial marking
b) Hibernation
c) Asexual reproduction
d) Solitary foraging

130. Altruistic behavior in animals is characterized by:

a) Selfish actions that benefit the individual
b) Actions that benefit other individuals at a cost to the actor
c) Competitive behavior within a group
d) Actions that benefit the individual without affecting others
b) Actions that benefit other individuals at a cost to the actor

131. Which of the following terms refers to a social hierarchy or ranking within a group of animals?

a) Eusociality
b) Dominance hierarchy
c) Territoriality
d) Matriarchy

132. Eusociality is a form of social organization seen in:

a) Solitary species
b) Highly social insects like ants and bees
c) Large herbivores
d) Arboreal primates

133. Which of the following is an example of mating systems commonly observed in social animals?
a) Monogamy
b) Asexuality
c) Herbivory
d) Parasitism

134. In social behavior, communication among animals can involve various signals, such as:
a) Emails and text messages
b) Chemical cues, vocalizations, and body language
c) Radar signals
d) Heat signatures

135. Which type of animal grouping is characterized by a temporary association of individuals, often for purposes such as foraging or predator avoidance?
a) Flock
b) Herd
c) Pack
d) Colony

136. Social behavior in animals can offer advantages, such as increased protection and resource sharing, but it may also involve competition and conflicts. Which of the following is an example of a potential disadvantage of social behavior?
a) Improved predator detection
b) Enhanced foraging efficiency
c) Increased risk of disease transmission
d) Better thermoregulation

137. What is the primary adaptive behavior observed in poultry regarding temperature regulation?
a) Sunbathing
b) Huddling
c) Swimming
d) Roosting

138. Which adaptive behavior do chickens exhibit when they detect a potential predator?
a) Camouflaging
b) Freezing
c) Flight response
d) Singing loudly

139. In response to changing daylight hours, many poultry species exhibit which adaptive behavior?
a) Migrating
b) Molting
c) Brooding
d) Seasonal reproduction

140. When a mother hen protects her chicks by spreading her wings and covering them, what is this behavior called?
a) Roosting
b) Brooding
c) Scratching
d) Grooming

141. Which adaptive behavior is associated with a male turkey displaying his colorful feathers and making sounds to attract a mate?
a) Nest building
b) Roosting
c) Strutting
d) Pecking

142. What is the adaptive behavior that allows poultry to find food by scratching the ground and using their beaks to search for insects and seeds?
 a) Nesting b) Foraging
 c) Sunbathing d) Preening
143. During extreme cold weather, poultry may exhibit what behavior to keep warm?
 a) Swimming b) Dust bathing
 c) Roosting d) Molting
144. Which adaptive behavior do ducks and geese engage in when they fly in a V-formation during migration?
 a) Sunbathing b) Roosting
 c) Nesting d) Flocking
145. What is the adaptive behavior that helps fish maintain buoyancy in water by adjusting their swim bladder's gas volume?
 a) Spawning b) Ovipositing
 c) Basking d) Buoyancy control
146. Many fish exhibit a daily migration pattern within the water column, moving to shallower waters at night and deeper waters during the day. What is this behavior called?
 a) Schooling b) Diel vertical migration
 c) Spawning d) Camouflage
147. Which adaptive behavior involves two or more fish swimming closely together in a coordinated manner for protection against predators and improved foraging opportunities?
 a) Camouflage b) Aggressive behavior
 c) Shoaling d) Ovipositing
148. Some fish species use this adaptive behavior to produce a temporary protective covering for their eggs:
 a) Spawning b) Nest-building
 c) Ovipositing d) Camouflage
149. What is the adaptive behavior where certain fish change their coloration and patterns to match their surroundings, making them less visible to predators and prey?
 a) Shoaling b) Spawning
 c) Camouflage d) Migratory behavior
150. Fish that engage in elaborate courtship rituals before mating often display which adaptive behavior?
 a) Schooling b) Ovipositing
 c) Aggressive behavior d) Spawning
151. Some fish, like salmon, exhibit an extraordinary adaptive behavior by returning to their natal streams to reproduce. What is this behavior called?
 a) Migratory behavior b) Buoyancy control
 c) Diel vertical migration d) Shoaling

152. What is the term for the adaptive behavior where fish engage in combat to establish dominance and access to resources within their territory?
   a) Spawning b) Camouflage
   c) Aggressive behavior d) Shoaling

153. What is the term for the innate behavior in reptiles that involves the use of sunlight or external heat sources to regulate body temperature?
   a) Hibernation b) Brumation
   c) Basking d) Migrating

154. Many reptiles, such as turtles and tortoises, display an innate behavior where they withdraw their limbs and head into their protective shell. What is this behavior called?
   a) Basking b) Camouflage
   c) Shell-gazing d) Retracting

155. Which innate behavior in reptiles refers to the shedding of their outer skin layer to accommodate growth and remove parasites?
   a) Basking b) Moulting
   c) Brumation d) Territorialism

156. Some reptiles, like snakes and certain lizards, exhibit an innate behavior of constriction when capturing prey. What is this behavior called?
   a) Ambushing b) Camouflage
   c) Constricting d) Slithering

157. Reptiles often engage in an innate behavior where they dig burrows and spend extended periods of dormancy in response to cold temperatures. What is this behavior called?
   a) Brumation b) Migrating
   c) Basking d) Slumbering

158. This innate behavior in reptiles involves the use of various body signals, such as head-bobbing, to communicate with potential rivals or mates:
   a) Moulting b) Ambushing
   c) Territory marking d) Ritualistic behavior

159. Some reptiles, like chameleons, display an innate behavior where they change the color of their skin to blend in with their environment or to communicate. What is this behavior called?
   a) Basking b) Camouflage
   c) Constricting d) Slithering

160. What is the term for the innate behavior in reptiles that involves the protective act of staying still and hidden to avoid detection by predators or prey?
   a) Ambushing b) Moulting
   c) Brumation d) Territorialism

Answer Key

1	b	2	c	3	a	4	c	5	a	6	a	7	a
8	d	9	a	10	b	11	b	12	d	13	c	14	b
15	c	16	a	17	c	18	a	19	b	20	a	21	a
22	c	23	b	24	c	25	a	26	d	27	b	28	a
29	a	30	a	31	d	32	d	33	d	34	a	35	c
36	c	37	d	38	a	39	c	40	a	41	a	42	a
43	b	44	c	45	c	46	d	47	a	48	b	49	d
50	b	51	d	52	c	53	c	54	b	55	c	56	d
57	c	58	c	59	c	60	c	61	b	62	c	63	c
64	d	65	a	66	a	67	c	68	a	69	b	70	b
71	c	72	c	73	b	74	a	75	c	76	c	77	c
78	b	79	d	80	b	81	c	82	c	83	c	84	b
85	c	86	b	87	d	88	c	89	c	90	c	91	c
92	b	93	a	94	d	95	c	96	c	97	b	98	c
99	b	100	c	101	b	102	c	103	c	104	b	105	b
106	b	107	d	108	b	109	c	110	d	111	c	112	c
113	d	114	b	115	a	116	b	117	c	118	c	119	a
120	b	121	b	122	d	123	c	124	c	125	b	126	b
127	c	128	c	129	b	130	c	131	b	132	a	133	a
134	b	135	a	136	c	137	b	138	c	139	d	140	b
141	c	142	b	143	c	144	d	145	d	146	b	147	c
148	b	149	c	150	d	151	d	152	c	153	c	154	d
155	b	156	c	157	a	158	d	159	b	160	a		

7

Movement and Migration

***Nikita Singh*[1], *Pramod Kumar*[2], *Rajesh Kumar*[1*] and *Bhoopendra Singh*[1]**

[1]Department of Veterinary Gynaecology and Obstetrics, College of Veterinary Science & Animal Husbandry, Acharya Narendra Deva University of Agriculture & Technology, Ayodhya, Uttar Pradesh

[2]Department of Veterinary Physiology and Biochemistry, College of Veterinary Science & Animal Husbandry, Acharya Narendra Deva University of Agriculture & Technology, Ayodhya, Uttar Pradesh

Introduction

From the tiniest insects to the largest blue whales, all species in the animal kingdom have been shown to undergo the migration. Millions of animals embark on epic journeys every year in search of food, shelter, and opportunity for mating. These animals routinely travel thousands of kilometres by land, sea, or air, which both tests and improves their endurance. Among the most striking animal migrations are those of Arctic terns. The long-distance migration of these little birds from pole to pole is well-known. They are thought to move over 40,000 kilometres (25,000 miles) a year, spending the majority of their time at sea chasing an endless summer. One of the most well-known migrations is that of the monarch butterfly, which travels across several generations. Though they are widespread throughout the United States and beyond, monarch butterflies are most known for their ability to travel 4,800 kilometres (3,000 miles) from Canada to Mexico. Millions of monarch butterflies fly south each year from their northern ranges to the oyamel fir forests near the Sierra Madre mountains, where they build massive roosts to remain warm throughout the winter. The monarchs begin their annual migration northwards in the spring, taking three to five generations to reach their goal. The migration that is the most dramatic belongs to the wildebeest. They coexist with thousands of zebras and gazelles in enormous herds that number over a million. The yearly migration of wildebeest across Tanzania and Kenya in quest of new water and grazing land is well-known. One of the most magnificent displays of nature is thought to be the migration. Animals that migrate are essential to preserving ecosystem balance and sustaining life as we know it. They distribute seeds and serve as pollinators, which support the structure and functionality of ecosystems. They maintain ecosystem balance by controlling the number of species and provide food for other creatures. Animals that migrate have the potential to be highly useful indicators of environmental changes that have an impact on all of us. Migratory animals also have a significant impact on local and global economies, as they provide food and revenue through subsistence, commercial and leisure hunting, and fishing. Furthermore, migratory animals are highly significant in many societies' myths, tales, religious doctrines, rituals, and medical practises. The way different animals prepare for migration is not always the same. Certain creatures, like birds, can navigate by using the positions of the sun and stars since they are born with a sense of direction. Some creatures, like monarch butterflies, use a variety of environmental signals to guide their migration, such as the sun's position, the Earth's magnetic field, and visible landmarks.

Migratory animals go through physiological changes before to setting off on their voyage, in order to prepare for the arduous trek ahead. For instance, in order to supply energy for their second flight, birds expand their fat reserves. Comparably, reproductive diapause is a process that monarch butterflies go through to save energy and postpone reproducing until they get to their destination. Animals that migrate have behavioural changes in addition to physiological ones. For instance, certain bird species separate into flocks prior to migration in order to lower their vulnerability to predators and improve their chances of obtaining food [2]. In a similar vein, several whale and dolphin species migrate in big groups in order to minimise drag and preserve energy.

All things considered, animals that migrate have developed a variety of pre-migration tactics that enable them to accomplish some of the most astounding things in the animal kingdom. Depending on the species, different animals can migrate over different distances. A study that was published in the journal Scientific Reports claims that caribou have the world's longest migrations, with round-trip durations of more than 745 miles (1,200 km). Nonetheless, records indicate that in year three, a Mongolian grey wolf covered a distance of more than 4,500 miles (7,247 kilometres). Animals that migrate use different navigational techniques based on their species. Certain creatures, like birds, can navigate by using the positions of the sun and stars because they have an innate sense of direction. Some creatures, like monarch butterflies, use a variety of environmental signals to guide their migration, such as the sun's position, the Earth's magnetic fields, and visible landmarks. Some creatures employ olfactory cues in addition to these ones for navigation; sea turtles, for instance, use them to find their nesting beaches.

MCQ's

1. For the public and for many biologists, the word migration evokes visions of "heroic" movements of whole populations over

   a) Short distance
   b) Long distance
   c) Both of the above
   d) None of the above

2. Migrating animals are found in all major branches of the animal kingdom, their journeys take place in a variety of media, and they move by-

   i) Flying
   ii) Swimming
   iii) Walking
   iv) Drifting

   a) i, ii, and iv are correct
   b) i, ii, iii and, iv are correct
   c) Only I and ii are correct
   d) Only iv is correct

3. Statement-1 Insects of the same or different generations may migrate several times within a breeding season,

   Statement-2 Fish such as herring may move in circuits between breeding, feeding, and wintering sites

   a) Only statement 1 is correct b) Only statement 1 is incorrect
   c) Both statements are incorrect d) Both statements are correct

4. Depending on whether they always migrate or do so only in a proximate response to current deterioration of local conditions migrants are often classified as either-

   a) Obligate b) Facultative
   c) Both d) None

5. In which type of migration, a fraction of the population remains either in its breeding or its nonbreeding area while the remainder moves away-

   a) In partial migration b) In complete migration
   c) In differential migration d) In all of the above

6. In which type of migration there are differences in the migration patterns of older and younger individuals or of the two sexes.

   a) In partial migration b) In complete migration
   c) In differential migration d) In all of the above

7. Migratory patterns is classifying as which of the following if the focus is on the organism-

   a) Obligate b) Facultative
   c) Partial and differential d) All of the above

8. Migratory patterns is classifying as which of the following if the focus is on the spatial or temporal attributes-

   a) To-and-fro
   b) One-way and Round-trip (loop)
   c) Altitudinal and nomadic
   d) All of the above

9. Migratory patterns is classifying as which of the following if the focus is on the medium in which migration takes place-

   a) Diadromic b) Drift (including devices)
   c) Both of the above d) None

10. Migratory patterns is classifying as which of the following if the focus is on the time at which migration takes place

    a) Seasonal b) Irruptive
    c) Both the above d) None of the above

11. Migration which we call here "two worlds" is

    a) To-and-fro b) One-way and Round-trip (loop)
    c) Altitudinal and nomadic d) All of the above

12. Which type of migration is a variant of to-and-fro migration in which animals return to the general breeding area from which they originated
    a) To-and-fro b) One-way and
    c) Altitudinal and nomadic d) Round-trip (loop)
13. One-way migrations, found mainly in-
    a) Insect larvae b) Marine larvae
    c) Mammals d) Both a and b
14. Migrations that occur between different water depths
    a) Diadromic b) Altitudinal
    c) Seasonal d) Vertical
15. Which migrations are actually a form of what we term "commuting"
    a) Diadromic b) Altitudinal
    c) Seasonal d) Vertical
16. Migrations that occur between different terrestrial elevations.
    a) Diadromic b) Altitudinal
    c) Seasonal d) Vertical
17. Migration does not follow a regular pattern or route but links temporary breeding sites that are located where conditions are ephemerally favourable.
    a) In Nomadism b) In Diadromic
    c) In Altitudinal d) In All
18. Which migrations are round trips synchronized with the annual cycle, and seasonal migrations are particular stages of these journeys.
    a) Annual migrations b) Daily migrations
    c) Seasonal migrations d) All of the above
19. Occasional, irregular movements of a significant proportion of a population beyond its usual breeding or nonbreeding area-
    a) Seasonal b) Irruptions
    c) Annual d) All of the above
20. Migrations encompasses all migratory movements between salt- and freshwater habitats, and is prevalent among fishes, with examples also from crustaceans and molluscs.
    a) Diadromic b) Altitudinal
    c) Seasonal d) Vertical
21. Migration occurs when animals migrate from freshwater to saltwater as adults, returning to freshwater to spawn
    a) Anadromy b) Catadromy
    c) Amphidromy d) All of the above
22. Situation in whichadults migrate to freshwater to feed and return to the ocean to spawn-
    a) Anadromy b) Catadromy
    c) Amphidromy d) All of the above

23. A form ofDiadromic whereby spawning can occur in either fresh- or saltwater, and where juveniles migrate to the alternative habitat to feed and grow and then return to their natal habitat to continue to feed and spawn-

    a) Anadromy
    b) Catadromy
    c) Amphidromy
    d) All of the above

24. Amphidromy that has been documented in a range of families, and is particularly prevalent among the sicydiine gobies-considered to be less widespread than-

    a) Anadromy
    b) Catadromy
    c) Both of the above
    d) None of the above

25. Assertion-Diadromy has been reported in just less than 1% of all fish species, but is of particular interest

    Reason- As many of these species are of commercial importance, such as the many anadromous salmonids

    a) Both Assertion (A) and Reason (R) are the true and Reason (R) is a correct explanation of Assertion (A)
    b) Both Assertion (A) and Reason (R) are the true but Reason (R) is not a correct explanation of Assertion (A).
    c) Assertion (A) is true and Reason (R) is false.
    d) Assertion (A) is false and Reason (R) is true.

26. Juvenile anadromous Pacific salmon can increase their growth rate by up to 50% in just the first week of life in

    a) The ocean
    b) The fresh water
    c) Both fresh and ocean water
    d) None of the above

27. Assertion- Anadromy is not more widespread.

    Reason-Estimates suggest that predation risk is significantly increased for oceanic migrants, and the energetic cost of migration itself can be very high in case of anadromy.

    a) Both Assertion (A) and Reason (R) are the true and Reason (R) is a correct explanation of Assertion (A).
    b) Both Assertion (A) and Reason (R) are the true but Reason (R) is not a correct explanation of Assertion (A) .
    c) Assertion (A) is true and Reason (R) is false.
    d) Assertion (A) is false and Reason (R) is true.

28. Assertion-Birds that breed in montane or moorland habitats, e.g. wallcreeper, Tichodroma muraria, and dipper, Cinclus spp., migrate to lower altitudes.

    Reason-To escape cold weather conditions at higher altitudes during winter.

    a) Both Assertion (A) and Reason (R) are the true and Reason (R) is a correct explanation of Assertion (A)
    b) Both Assertion (A) and Reason (R) are the true but Reason (R) is not a correct explanation of Assertion (A)
    c) Assertion (A) is true and Reason (R) is false
    d) Assertion (A) is false and Reason (R) is true

29. Identify the landscape barriers-
    i) Mountain ranges ii) Rivers
    iii) Deserts
    a) i, and ii, are correct b) ii and iii are correct
    c) Only i is correct d) All are correct answers
30. Assertion- Landscape barriers can have major impacts upon ecological processes
    Reason- Their disruptive effect upon animal movements such as migration and dispersal.
    a) Both Assertion (A) and Reason (R) are the true and Reason (R) is a correct explanation of Assertion (A).
    b) Both Assertion (A) and Reason (R) are the true but Reason (R) is not a correct explanation of Assertion (A).
    c) Assertion (A) is true and Reason (R) is false.
    d) Assertion (A) is false and Reason (R) is true
31. Many terrestrial migrants migrate along relatively predictable routes, as-
    a) Along valleys
    b) Ridges in mountainous regions
    c) Both of the above
    d) None of the above
32. Anthropogenic developments that had impacts upon migration and migratory routes for many speciesand have changed the landscape topography are-
    a) Pipelines b) Train tracks,
    c) Roads, and urbanization d) All of the above
33. Assertion-In particular, many studies have assessed the impact of barriers arising from the rapid expansion of transport infrastructure that has fragmented terrestrial ecosystems worldwide.
    Reason- These studies have documented that roads railroads, and their traffic disrupt animal migration and ecological processes, and also increase mortality and lead to habitat degradation, loss, and isolation.
    a) Both Assertion (A) and Reason (R) are the true and Reason (R) is a correct explanation of Assertion (A).
    b) Both Assertion (A) and Reason (R) are the true but Reason (R) is not a correct explanation of Assertion (A).
    c) Assertion (A) is true and Reason (R) is false.
    d) Assertion (A) is false and Reason (R) is true
34. Roads have a number of ecological effects, but perhaps the most damaging is the disruption they cause to-
    a) Animal movement b) Animal feeding
    c) Animal predations d) None of the above

35. Which anthropogenic infrastructure can be severe enough to cause genetic differentiation between populations on either side of the barrier-

a) Pipelines
b) Roads
c) Urbanization
d) None

36. Identify the correct one regarding Habitat fragmentation in freshwater in form of natural features are such as-

i) Sandbars
ii) Landslides
iii) Waterfalls
iv) Boulder cascades
v) Roads and Dam

a) Only i, ii, and iv are correct
b) Only i, iii and, iv are correct
c) Only iv and v are incorrect
d) Only v is incorrect

37. Read the statements carefully-

Statement 1- Many dams provide no mechanism for adult fish to pass above the dam, thus blocking off spawning habitat upstream.

Statement 2- When fish passages do exist, many migratory fish have trouble finding the fish ladders on dams or die when exposed to higher water temperatures inside the ladders.

Statement 3- Even if the fish manage to find the ladders and survive the arduous journey to their spawning grounds, individuals are often too exhausted from the journey to spawn successfully.

a) Only statement 1 is correct
b) Only statement 1 is incorrect
c) Only Statements 2 is incorrect
d) All statements are correct

38. Marine systems are generally considered more homogenous than-

a) Terrestrial environment
b) Freshwater environment
c) Areal environment
d) Both a and c

39. Assertion- Ocean currents and environmental gradients do not pose a barrier to all animals

Reason- Some animals might even adopt behavioural strategies to use surface water currents during long-distance travel, enabling them to move quickly and efficiently over considerable distances.

a) Both Assertion (A) and Reason (R) are the true and Reason (R) is a correct explanation of Assertion (A).
b) Both Assertion (A) and Reason (R) are the true but Reason (R) is not a correct explanation of Assertion (A).
c) Assertion (A) is true and Reason (R) is false.
d) Assertion (A) is false and Reason (R) is true

40. Amphibians and terrestrial crabs are prone to desiccation and during migration require access to-

a) Dry and Desert
b) Water or Wet conditions
c) Humidity
d) All of the above

41. Many ungulates may track the routes along the migratory journey which have
    a) 'Green wave' of forage b) Dry wave of forage
    c) Water and river range d) All of the above
42. The patter of migratory behaviour are-
    a) Static b) Variable
    c) More static less variable d) All of the above
43. Many migratory species are now in decline due to-
    a) Habitat loss b) Exploitation
    c) Damming d) All of the above
44. Statement 1-Climate change can also influence the fitness outcomes of migrants and residents in partially migratory populations, and thus alter population patterns of migratory behaviour.

    Statement 2- In partially anadromous fishes, human exploitation can act as a powerful selective force against migratory behaviour, as can the damming of rivers.
    a) Only statement 1 is correct b) Only statement 1 is incorrect
    c) Only Statements 2 is incorrect d) All statements are correct
45. The migration of which taxa requires little more than a minor extension of typical physiological characteristics-
    a) Mammalian b) Mollusca
    c) Insects d) Fishes
46. Almost without exception, even outside of the migration seasonmigratory mammals are highly-
    a) Very much stationary b) Mobile
    c) Immobile d) All of the above
47. Assertion- mammal migration differs markedly from avian, fish, or insect migrations.

    Reason-In these species mobility often increases by an order of magnitude when entering the migratory phase.
    a) Both Assertion (A) and Reason (R) are the true and Reason (R) is a correct explanation of Assertion (A).
    b) Both Assertion (A) and Reason (R) are the true but Reason (R) is not a correct explanation of Assertion (A).
    c) Assertion (A) is true and Reason (R) is false
    d) Assertion (A) is false and Reason (R) is true
48. The knowledge of successful migrant needs to "know" when to leave its current range, where to move, and when to stop, may be transferred-
    a) Genetically inherited b) Culturally
    c) Behaviourally d) Both a and b

49. Read the statements carefully regarding themode fortransferring the knowledge of migration in a member of species with in single generation or one generation to another generation-

Statement 1- A study of zebra (Equus burchelli) in Botswana recorded migratory movements retracing a historical migratory route that had been blocked by fences during the previous 36 years prior to the study

Statement 2- As culturally transferred knowledge is unlikely over such an extended period, these findings suggest that zebra migration has at least some genetically inherited component

Statement 3-Alternatively, exploratory behaviour could have encouraged rapid identification of fitness improving patterns of range use once the barrier was removed, allowing zebra to rapidly "re-learn" a culturally transmitted trait.

a) Only statement 1 and 2are correct
b) Only statement 1 is incorrect
c) Only Statements 3 is incorrect
d) All statements are correct

50. In avian migration, it is fairly common to observe complex migratory networks with a mixture of multiple-

a) Wintering sites
b) Breeding sites
c) Both a and b
d) None of the above

51. Ungulate migratory routes along river valleys can be quite narrow, and therefore vulnerable to inadvertent creation of barriers, such as from-

i) Oil wells
ii) Housing developments
iii) Anthropogenic environmental modifications

a) Only i, ii, are correct
b) Only iii is correct
c) Only i is incorrect
d) All are correct

52. Statement 1-Maintaining the integrity of migratory networks would seem one of the most important conservation needs.

Statement 2-Unlike other taxa, long-distance migration in most mammals probably requires only minor phenotypic modification in body plan.

a) Only statement 1 is correct
b) Only statement 1 is incorrect
c) Both Statements are incorrect
d) Both statements are correct

53. In which speciesMigratory networks are thought to have a strong suppressive effect on local adaptations because of substantial gene flow among subpopulations

a) In mammals
b) In birds
c) In reptiles
d) In amphibians

54. Migration is well developed among ungulates of orders-

a) Perissodactyla (odd-toed)
b) Artiodactyla (even-toed)
c) Both of the above
d) None of the above

55. Ungulates may also benefit from reduced predation pressure while-

a) Free grazing
b) Migrating
c) Drinking near the pond
d) All of the above

56. Assertion- Resident populations of Himalayan tahr (Hemitragus jemlahicus) exhibit fluctuating seasonal abundance of males,

Reason- Sexual differences in nutritional demands often produces seasonal patterns of sexual segregation in ungulates

a) Both Assertion (A) and Reason (R) are the true and Reason (R) is a correct explanation of Assertion (A).

b) Both Assertion (A) and Reason (R) are the true but Reason (R) is not a correct explanation of Assertion (A).

c) Assertion (A) is true and Reason (R) is false.

d) Assertion (A) is false and Reason (R) is true

57. Migration is decidedly common in which whales-

a) Toothed (Odontoceti) whales b) Baleen (Mysticeti) whales

c) Both a and b d) None of the above

58. Migratory behaviourof whale is primarily influenced by seasonal trade-offs between optimal environmental conditions for-

a) Breeding b) Feeding

c) Wandering d) Both a and b

59. Tropical waters favoured for whale-calf thermoregulation during which season-

a) Winter b) Summer

c) Spring d) Rainy season

60. Arctic regions favouredwhales because of dramatic increase in food availability during the

a) Winter and spring b) Summer and winter

c) Spring and summer d) Winter and monsoon

61. Hump back whales reliably breed at approximately 20° latitude regardless of hemisphere, then return to subarctic waters to feed after fasting throughout the-

a) Breeding season b) Growing season

c) Both a and b d) None of the above

62. Which type of migration is decidedly common across all migratory cetaceans

a) Partial migration

b) Complete migration

c) Some time partial but mostly complete migration

d) All of the above

63. Partial migration in cetaceans is frequently linked to sexual differences in

a) Only nutrition b) Only parental care

c) Nutrition and parental care both d) Environmental conditions

64. Female and juvenile bowhead whales may use alternate southward migratory routes compared with-

a) Male bowhead whales

b) Other female bowhead whales

c) Both male as well as female bowhead male
d) None of these

65. The migratory behavior of bats seems to be primarily driven by seasonality, due to changes in-
a) Abiotic environmental conditions
b) Resource availability
c) Genetic variance
d) Both a & b

66. The migratory behavior seems to be primarily driven by seasonality is particularly true for bats occurring in which climates-
a) Temperate
b) Tropical
c) Tundra
d) All of the above

67. Mainly whichspecies of bataresuffering extreme variation in resource abundance due to plant phenology and are therefore expected to undergo seasonal range shifts that track shifting spatial inflorescence patterns
a) Frugivorous
b) Nectivorous
c) Omnivorous
d) Both a & b

68. In numerous species of bats, migratory behavior differs substantially-
a) Between populations
b) Within populations
c) Between and within populations
d) Never differ in any way

69. Statement 1- It is noteworthy that bat migratory behavior is heavily influence by wing morphology.

Statement2- Migratory bats often possess wings adapted to long-distance travel: long and narrow, with decidedly pointed wing tips
a) Only statement 1is correct
b) Only statement 1 is incorrect
c) Only Statements 2 is incorrect
d) Both statements are correct

70. The wing adaptations in batrestrict in-flight manoeuvrability, however, limiting the capacity to-
a) Hover and travel with fast velocities
b) Hover and travel at low velocities
c) Travel with combination of velocities
d) None of the above

71. Migration in many bats may therefore be a secondary benefit of specific morphological adaptations enhancing-
a) Foraging success
b) Easy movements
c) Reproduction quality
d) None of the above

72. Read the statements carefully and identify the correct one-

Statement 1- Seasonal movements of elephants coincide with rainfall patterns.

Statement 2- Elephants do not typically migrate between predictable areas or regions.

Statement 3-Elephants migrate between predictable habitat types.
a) Only statement 1 and 2 are correct
b) Only statement 1 is incorrect
c) Only Statements 3 is incorrect
d) All statements are correct

73. Read the points regarding African elephant migration and identify the correct points-

 i) They track primary productivity and forage quality as influenced by rainfall

 ii) Often moving into forested habitat during the dry season to mate and rear young

 iii) Returning to more open foraging areas when primary productivity increases at the onset of the rainy season.

 iv) Such migrations rarely involve the entire population, often being limited to family units.

 a) Only i, ii and iv, are correct b) Only iii is incorrect

 c) Only I and iv is incorrect d) All are correct

74. Elephant family units regularly between Uganda and Sudan, and accounts suggest that they may travel from Mount Kilimanjaro to the Lorian Swamp in Kenya and back,the traveling distance are respectively-

 a) 160 km & 480–640 km b) 480-650 km & 160 km

 c) 750 km & 990 – 1000 km d) 990- 1000 km & 750 km

75. Members of order carnivora often establish and maintain or defend territories for the purposes of hunting and mating, which precludes the possibility of-

 a) Shelter b) Migration

 c) Immigration d) Emigration

76. All extant families of suborder Pinnipedia (walruses, Odobenidae; eared seals, Otariidae; earless seals, Phocidae) contain at least how much migratory species-

 a) Thousands b) Hundreds

 c) Tens d) One

77. In seals, migratory behavior often coincides with distinct foraging and breeding areas (i.e., rookeries), as in-

 a) Southern elephant seals b) Northern elephant seals.

 c) Northern fur seals and harp seals d) All of the above

78. Both extant genera of order Sirenia, first manatees and dugongs are-

 a) Migratory b) None migratory

 c) Only sometimes migratory d) All of the above

79. Movements by Amazonian and African manatees are seemingly influenced by seasonal changes in water depth, effectively trading off areas of high resource density vs. low predation pressure that are used equally by-

 a) Male population b) Female population

 c) Both sexes d) Hermaphrodites

80. West Indian manatees often follow a north–south migration route based on water temperature and exhibit sexual differences in-

 a) Migration velocity b) Migration direction

 c) Site preference d) both a and c

81. Dugongs follow migratory patterns similar to those of manatees: at which latitudes (e.g., southern Australia) dugong populations tend to track seasonal changes in water temperature, whereas dugongs at which latitudes typically respond to changes in water depth and the hydrological cycle respectively

a) High, low b) High, high
c) Low, high d) Low, low

82. The lone migratory species of *Lagomorpha*order which migrates to distinct wintering grounds southwest of its normal feeding grounds is-

a) White-tailed jack-rabbit b) Black-tailed jack-rabbit
c) Brown-tailed jack-rabbit d) Golden-tailed jack-rabbit

83. Statement 1- There is anecdotal evidence to suggest that gorillas (*Gorilla gorilla*) never use regular migration routes while searching for foraging grounds

Statement 2- the majority of literature on primate migration describes emigration–immigration of individuals between groups and semi-nomadism.

a) Only statement 1 is correct b) Only statement 1 is incorrect
c) Only Statements 2 is incorrect d) All statements are correct

84. Statement 1-Migration was a well-developed life-history strategy in several different preindustrial human societies.

Statement 2- Several Indian tribes living on the Great Plains of North America relied on the Plains bison for a large fraction of their meat protein.

a) Only statement 1 is correct b) Only statement 1 is incorrect
c) Only Statements 2 is incorrect d) All statements are correct

85. The Sioux were particularly renowned for their ability to track buffalo migrations for extended periods, developing an entire economy around-

a) Bison-derived goods b) Cattle-derived goods
c) Yak-derived goods d) All are correct

86. Statement 1- Inuit people in the areas fringing the Arctic Ocean also migrated from inland areas occupied during the winter to the seaside during the brief summer.

Statement 2- This will not allow Inuit people to take maximum advantage of the rich assortment of fish and sea mammals available in Arctic waters during the ice-free period, but shifting back onto the tundra to hunt caribou, moose, and other terrestrial mammals during the winter.

Statement 3- Similar migrations are well documented across Siberia.

a) Only statement 1 and 2 are correct b) Only statement 1 is incorrect
c) Only Statements 2 is incorrect d) All statements are correct

87. Pastoralist societies often migrated with their herds in a manner remarkably similar to that of-

a) Wild ungulates b) Domesticated ungulates
c) Both a & b d) None

88. Assertion- The most prominent exception is terrestrial carnivores, among which there are relatively few true migrants.

Reason- The reasons for this are rather unclear, but likely stem from spatial restrictions imposed by social structure, such as territoriality and exclusive home-range use.

a) Both Assertion (A) and Reason (R) are the true and Reason (R) is a correct explanation of Assertion (A).

b) Both Assertion (A) and Reason (R) are the true but Reason (R) is not a correct explanation of Assertion (A).

c) Assertion (A) is true and Reason (R) is false.

d) Assertion (A) is false and Reason (R) is true

89. Statement 1- There is also growing evidence that herbivore migration can reduce predation risk, at least in systems with top carnivores with territorial social systems.

Statement 2- Among mammalian carnivores, variation in food quality is undoubtedly a minor concern because their prey species are nutritionally identical to themselves, at least in a crude sense.

a) Only statement 1 is correct b) Only statement 1 is incorrect

c) Only Statements 2 is correct d) Both statements are correct

90. There seem to be two alternative pathways to the evolution of migration.

i) First, some terrestrial predators have seemingly evolved the ability to migrate to track their migratory prey.

ii) Second, aquatic predators seem to trade off energetic costs against benefits of feeding in resource-rich environments

a) Only pathway 1 is correct b) Only pathway 1 is incorrect

c) Only pathway 2 is correct d) Both pathways are correct

91. Why do we need to understand patterns of movement of wild animals.

a) For understanding their ecology b) Life history and behavior

c) Effective conservation d) All of the above

92. To track a diversity of animal species in a variety of habitats we use-

a) Unstable isotope marker b) Stable isotope markers

c) Radioactivemarker d) All of the above

93. We use the stable isotopes for tracking purposeby making connections between phases of the annual cycle of-

a) Migratory animals b) Non migratory animals

c) Immigrants d) All of the above

94. Which of the following markers used to track animal movements is extrinsic in nature.

a) Genetic variation b) Remote sensing

c) Stable isotopes d) Behavioural variation

95. Analyse the below statements and choose the appropriate option.

Statement 1- Stable isotopes are intrinsic markers.

Statement 2- Stable isotopes are extrinsic markers.

Statement 3- Intrinsic markers are used to infer geographical origins and to differentiate among populations of animals.

a) 1 and 3 are correct b) 2 and 3 are correct

c) Only 1 is incorrect d) All are correct

96. The marker which do not require marking or recapturing individual animals-

a) Chemical markers b) Biogeochemical markers

c) Environmental markers d) Genetic markers

97. Which of the following method suffers with 'needle-in-a-haystack' effect?

a) Extrinsic marker b) Biological marker

c) Biogeochemical marker d) Environmentalmarker

98. What is the limitation of biological markers?

a) Relies heavily on capturing specific individuals

b) Seasonal migration

c) It works well over geographical scales of thousands of kilometres

d) None of the above

99. Assertion: Stable isotopes behave differently in biogeochemical processes

Reason: Stable isotopes are naturally occurring stable forms of elements with differing nuclear masses, which confer disparate physical properties

a) Both Assertion (A) and Reason (R) are the true and Reason (R) is a correct explanation of Assertion (A)

b) Both Assertion (A) and Reason (R) are the true but Reason (R) is not a correct explanation of Assertion (A)

c) Assertion (A) is true and Reason (R) is false

d) Assertion (A) is false and Reason (R) is true

100. Stable isotopes are used in ecological studies primarily to:

a) Determine the age of animals

b) Assess the reproductive rates of populations

c) Study the genetics

d) Stable isotopes are incorporated directly through diet into animal tissues

101. Which of the following is a light isotope.

a) Strontium b) Sulphur

c) Lead d) Cerium

102. Which is defined as a change in position of an individual in time, has been studied at least since classical antiquity, both from conceptual *(Aristotle's De motu animalium 384-322 Bc* and mechanistic *(Galen's De motu musculorum 129-210 AD)* perspectives.

a) Movement
b) Migration
c) Mutation
d) All of the above

103. In recent years, the technological and analytical advances for animal and human tracking triggered the emergence of a series of reviews to study different aspects of movement ecology are-

a) Related to sensors
b) Software
c) Statistical
d) Mathematical tools
a) a and b are correct
b) c and d are correct
c) Only d is incorrect
d) All are correct

104. Improvements in technological devices to track animals and humans have generated high volumes of movement data from a range of species, providing greater information on their-

a) Movement paths
b) Physiology
c) Environment they experience
d) All of the above

105. Not all round trips are necessarily repeated on an annual basis and for some animal's migration and subsequent breeding actually coincides with death, a phenomenon known as-

a) Semelparous migration
b) Altitudinal migration
c) Spatial migration
d) Both a and c

106. Most insects do not survive long enough to make a return journey during a seasonal migration cycle. A number of lepidopterans have evolved an unusual response to this problem, known as-

a) Transgenerational migration
b) Semelparous migration
c) Spatial migration
d) All of the above

107. Read the statements carefully -

Statements 1- There is a great diversity of patterns of migratory timing in the animal kingdom.

Statements 2- Migratory timing may be highly synchronized, such as is the case with the mass migration of Christmas Island red crabs

Statements 3- The degree of synchrony can vary depending on season

a) 1 and 3 are correct
b) 2 and 3 are correct
c) Only 1 is incorrect
d) All are correct

108. Migratorysynchronization may be

i) Active, i.e. due to benefits that can be accrued due to migrating in mass such as a dilution effect versus predators (*Krause and Ruxton 2002*), or in order to maximize reproductive success.

ii) Passive, and driven by exogenous cues shared by many individuals of the same species, such as photoperiod.

a) i and ii are incorrect
b) Only ii is incorrect
c) Only i is incorrect
d) All are correct

109. If we are to successfully conserve the vast biological diversity that encompasses the myriad migratory species, understanding the broader patterns of migration is-
a) Essential
b) Nonessential
c) Sometime essential
d) All of the above

110. Assertion-In a changing world, patterns of migration are not static, but can shift in step with the environment in many cases.

Reason-If migrants are unable to adapt to environmental changes along the migratory route, they are also at risk of population declines and potential extirpation.
a) Both Assertion (A) and Reason (R) are the true and Reason (R) is a correct explanation of Assertion (A).
b) Both Assertion (A) and Reason (R) are the true but Reason (R) is not a correct explanation of Assertion (A).
c) Assertion (A) is true and Reason (R) is false.
d) Assertion (A) is false and Reason (R) is true

111. Given the taxonomic breadth of migration it is perhaps no surprise that the phenomenon is so wonderfully-
a) Heterogenous
b) Homogenous
c) More homogenous less heterogenous
d) All of the above

112. International Union for Conservation of Nature (IUCN) Red List suggests that mobile species are not more likely to be classified as globally threatened and are not being added to the IUCN Red List at a faster rate than -(Kirby *et al.* 2008).
a) Sedentary species
b) Mountain mobile species
c) Rapid mobile species
d) All of the above

113. Assertion-observed rapid declines in mobile species around the world (Kirby *et al.* 2008)

Reason- this above decline rate suggest that time is running out to achieve the large-scale conservation action necessary to avert the loss of these great wildlife spectacles.
a) Both Assertion (A) and Reason (R) are the true and Reason (R) is a correct explanation of Assertion (A).
b) Both Assertion (A) and Reason (R) are the true but Reason (R) is not a correct explanation of Assertion (A).
c) Assertion (A) is true and Reason (R) is false.
d) Assertion (A) is false and Reason (R) is true

114. Migration involves a complex, interrelated suite of physiological, morphological and behavioural traits that are mediated by an inherited 'migratory gene package', which in turn can be viewed as part of a-

a) Migratory syndrome b) Mutational syndrome

c) Genomic syndrome d) None of the above

115. Migratory adaptations arise and vanish-

a) Rapidly b) Slowly

c) Moderately d) None

116. Long-distance migration imposes severe demands on the-

a) Pathology of the animals b) Physiology of animals

c) Genomics of the animals d) None of the above

117. An interesting set of adaptations enables migratory birds to accumulate enormous fat stores, up to-

a) 50–60% of body mass b) 80-90% of body mass

c) 10-20% of body mass d) b and c are correct

118. Fat storage and then transport and oxidize fatty acids at a sufficiently high rate to sustain constant activity of which muscles over days or weeks.

a) Flight muscles b) Brest muscles

c) Thigh muscles d) All of the above

119. Some migrants engage in preferentially selecting favourable foods that enhance migratory performance which is known as-

a) Natural adaptation b) Natural selection

c) Natural doping d) Natural mutation

120. Statement 1- metabolism and energetics are not the only factors that make longdistance migration possible.

Statement 2- No single physiological adaptation transforms an animal into an endurance specialist.

a) Only i is correct b) Only ii is correct

c) Both are incorrect d) Both are correct

121. Factors contributing to the decline of migrants include-

i) Climate change, ii) Overexploitation,

iii) Barriers, iv) Habitat destruction,

v) Fatalities from unintended anthropogenic interactions, such as fisheries bycatch or fatal collisions with wind turbinesand vehicles

a) Only ii and iii are incorrect b) Only iv and v is incorrect

c) Only i, iii andv is correct d) All are correct

122. Migration, in particular, affects biodiversity at regional and global scales, and migratory animals affect-

a) Ecosystem processes b) Physiological processes

c) Behavioural processes d) All of the above

123. Animals use predictable environmental cues for the timing and navigation of migration. A change in these cues will affect the migration by mean of-
   a) Phenology
   b) Extent
   c) Both phenology and extent of migration
   d) None of the above

124. Which one in the following is phenological markers in migrating birds-
   a) Arrival date
   b) Hatching date
   c) Both arrival and hatching dates
   d) None of the above

125. Assertion- Arrival date and hatching date in migrating birds can be strongly affected by global warming.

   Reason- Higher temperatures cause earlier appearance of the insect prey of hatchling birds, which exerts pressure on birds to breed earlier so that hatchling development coincides with peak prey abundance.
   a) Both Assertion (A) and Reason (R) are the true and Reason (R) is a correct explanation of Assertion (A).
   b) Both Assertion (A) and Reason (R) are the true but Reason (R) is not a correct explanation of Assertion (A).
   c) Assertion (A) is true and Reason (R) is false.
   d) Assertion (A) is false and Reason (R) is true

126. Phenological shifts in migration of endothermic birds are linked to the abundance of their-
   a) Endothermic prey
   b) Ectothermic prey
   c) Mesothermic prey
   d) All of the above

127. At which extreme temperatures, cessation of physiological functions leads to mortality-
   a) Extreme low
   b) Extreme high
   c) Both extreme low and extreme high
   d) None can cause mortality

128. If fish did not have to replenish metabolic substrates (in particular glycogen) during their migration, the effects of warm water could be mitigated by swimming through warm sections of river at which rate-
   a) Rapidly
   b) Slowly
   c) Moderately
   d) Very slow

129. Assertion- Similar to birds, a recent study has shown that the phenology of migration of aphids in the UK has changed as a result of climate change

Reason- Seven hundred seventy trap-years of data collected over the past 50 years showed that over 55 species of aphids started flying progressively earlier in the year, and most species showed increasing duration of their flying season

a) Both Assertion (A) and Reason (R) are the true and Reason (R) is a correct explanation of Assertion (A).

b) Both Assertion (A) and Reason (R) are the true but Reason (R) is not a correct explanation of Assertion (A).

c) Assertion (A) is true and Reason (R) is false.

d) Assertion (A) is false and Reason (R) is true

130. To determine the thermal sensitivity of, for example, cardiovascular function and metabolism experimentally, it is possible to use these data to predict the effects of-

a) Future change
b) Regional climatic change
c) Future or regional climate change
d) none of the above

131. Statement 1- A new study now shows that changes in migratory behaviour also alter the incidence of infectious disease and its transmission.

Statement2- In addition to shifts in phenology of migrating animals, some species have reduced their migratory behaviour or even formed sedentary populations as a result of anthropogenic changes to the environment.

a) Only i is correct
b) Only ii is correct
c) All are incorrect
d) All are correct

132. Assertion- Migration can reduce the incidence of disease.

Reason-Because individuals leave contaminated habitats periodically, individuals are more separated from each other during migration, and infected individuals are likely to succumb to demanding long-distance movement.

a) Both Assertion (A) and Reason (R) are the true and Reason (R) is a correct explanation of Assertion (A).

b) Both Assertion (A) and Reason (R) are the true but Reason (R) is not a correct explanation of Assertion (A).

c) Assertion (A) is true and Reason (R) is false.

d) Assertion (A) is false and Reason (R) is true.

133. Assertion- Monarch butterflies in the US have drastically changed their migratory behaviour in recent years.

Reason-due to result of habitat alterations, and the incidence of sedentary, non-migratory populations is increasing.

a) Both Assertion (A) and Reason (R) are the true and Reason (R) is a correct explanation of Assertion (A).

b) Both Assertion (A) and Reason (R) are the true but Reason (R) is not a correct explanation of Assertion (A).

c) Assertion (A) is true and Reason (R) is false.

d) Assertion (A) is false and Reason (R) is true

134. Assertion-Nonmigratory butterflies have significantly reduced lifespan.

Reason- Nonmigratory populations have a significantly greater rate of infection by the protozoan *Ophryocystis elektroscirrha* compared to migratory populations.

a) Both Assertion (A) and Reason (R) are the true and Reason (R) is a correct explanation of Assertion (A).

b) Both Assertion (A) and Reason (R) are the true but Reason (R) is not a correct explanation of Assertion (A).

c) Assertion (A) is true and Reason (R) is false.

d) Assertion (A) is false and Reason (R) is true

135. Changes in animal movement and migration as a result of habitat modification and climate change may therefore alter lifetime fitness of individuals in addition to biodiversity and ecosystem processes at which scales.

a) Regional scale b) Global scale

c) Both regional and global scale d) None of the above

136. Which regions are experiencing the most rapid climate and environmental changes on Earth, caused primarily by anthropogenic greenhouse gas emissions.

a) Asiatic and adjacent b) Antarctic and adjacent

c) Arctic and adjacent d) All of the above

137. Assertion- The timing of parturition is a key to the demography of wildlife populations and can be an adaptive response to climate shifts.

Reason- For many mammals, the period from late pregnancy through weaning has the highest energetic demands and thus is timed to occur when vegetation productivity is highest

a) Both Assertion (A) and Reason (R) are the true and Reason (R) is a correct explanation of Assertion (A).

b) Both Assertion (A) and Reason (R) are the true but Reason (R) is not a correct explanation of Assertion (A).

c) Assertion (A) is true and Reason (R) is false.

d) Assertion (A) is false and Reason (R) is true

138. The southern and northern boreal populations calved earliest, followed by-

a) Northern mountain populations

b) Southern mountain populations

c) Northern and southern mountain populations

d) Western mountain populations

139. All species exhibited lower movement rates during winter relative to-

a) Spring b) Summer

c) Extreme winter d) All of the above

140. Migratory species are widespread in terrestrial, aquatic and aerial environments, and are important-

a) Ecologically b) Economically

c) Both ecologically and economically d) None of the above

141. The current understanding of migration indicates that-

Statement 1-Drivers of migration vary across species and ecosystems.

Statement 2- A species ability to adapt to environmental change successfully depends in part on its migration drivers.

a) Only i is correct b) Only ii is correct

c) Only i is incorrect d) All are correct

142. The inheritance process involves neither a single nor a dominant gene, but rather that migrating and not migrating are under-

a) Under polygenic control b) Quantitative genetic traits

c) Under qualitative genetic traits d) Both a and b

143. By which year a further global warming amounting to 1.4-5.8 □is predicted (Berthold, 1998; Kerr, 2001).

a) 2100 b) 4100

c) 5100 d) 5500

144. Global warming results are becoming evident; as-

i) The onset of spring at higher latitudes has advanced by at least a week,

ii) Glaciers and parts of the polar ice caps have receded,

iii) The sea level has risen.

iv) Mountains becoming more high

a) Only i, and iiiare correct b) Only ii, iii and ivare correct

c) Only iv is incorrect d) All are correct

145. There is evidence indicating the existence of an innate migratory drive as well as genetic control of-

i) The onset, duration and end of the migration period,

ii) The amount of migratory activity, a genetically prescribed parameter that determines the distance over which the bird flies.

iii) The migration directions

iv) Physiological parameters, in particular fat deposition during the migratory period

a) Only i and iv are correct b) Only ii is incorrect

c) Only i, ii, and ivare correct d) All are correct

146. A theory postulates that even in forms that at present are exclusively migratory, selection for lower levels of migratory activity can cause a threshold to be crossed, below which nonmigrants appear it is a-

a) New bird migration theory b) Old bird migration theory

c) Universal theory on bird's migration d) All of the above

147. Conversion of a population from migratory to nonmigratory can occur by selection with a transition through partial migration. This intermediate stage is prevalent among the-

a) Old bird species b) Recent bird species

c) Both a and b d) Not apply on bird species

148. Assertion- In current scenario migration an endangered phenomenon.

Reason- Around the world, many of the most spectacular migrations have either disappeared due to human activities or are in steep decline.

a) Both Assertion (A) and Reason (R) are the true and Reason (R) is a correct explanation of Assertion (A).

b) Both Assertion (A) and Reason (R) are the true but Reason (R) is not a correct explanation of Assertion (A).

c) Assertion (A) is true and Reason (R) is false.

d) Assertion (A) is false and Reason (R) is true

149. Those of us living in eastern North America can no longer experience the flocks of millions of which birds that temporarily obscured the sun as they migrated to and from their breeding grounds.

a) Passenger pigeons
b) Zooplanktons
c) Flamingos
d) Ostriches

150. In central Asia, the number of saiga, a peculiar migratory antelope of the dry steppe grasslands and semidesert, has dropped by-

i) Over 95% in the past two decades,

ii) Over one million to fewer than 50,000

a) Only i is correct
b) Only ii is correct
c) Both i and ii are incorrect
d) Both i and ii are correct

151. The causes of declines in migrates vary depending on the species and the locale, but in general, the threats to migrants fall into four nonexclusive categories: habitat destruction, the creation of obstacles and barriers such as-

a) Dams and fences
b) Overexploitation,
c) Climate change
d) All of the above

Answer Key

1	b	2	b	3	d	4	c	5	a	6	c	7	d
8	d	9	c	10	c	11	a	12	d	13	d	14	d
15	d	16	b	17	a	18	a	19	b	20	a	21	a
22	b	23	c	24	c	25	a	26	a	27	a	28	a
29	d	30	a	31	c	32	d	33	b	34	a	35	b
36	d	37	d	38	d	39	a	40	b	41		42	b
43	d	44	d	45	a	46	b	47	a	48	d	49	d
50	c	51	d	52	d	53	b	54	c	55	b	56	a
57	c	58	d	59	a	60	c	61	a	62	a	63	c
64	a	65	d	66	a	67	d	68	c	69	d	70	b
71	a	72	d	73	d	74	a	75	b	76	d	77	a
78	a	79	c	80	d	81	a	82	b	83	b	84	d
85	a	86	c	87	a	88	a	89	d	90	d	91	d

92	b	93	a	94	b	95	a	96	b	97	a	98	c
99	a	100	d	101	b	102	a	103	d	104	d	105	a
106	a	107	d	108	d	109	a	110	b	111	a	112	a
113	b	114	a	115	a	116	b	117	a	118	a	119	c
120	d	121	d	122	a	123	c	124	c	125	b	126	b
127	c	128	a	129	b	130	c	131	d	132	a	133	a
134	a	135	c	136	c	137	b	138	c	139	b	140	c
141	d	142	d	143	a	144	c	145	d	146	a	147	b
148	a	149	a	150	d	151	d						

8

Orientation, Navigation and Communication

Chetna Mahajan[1], Abhishek Gupta[2] and M.P.S. Tomar[3]

[1]*Guru Angad Dev Veterinary & Animal Sciences University, Ludhiana*

[2]*Rajasthan University of Veterinary & Animal Sciences, Bikaner*

Introduction

Animals have evolved various sophisticated methods for orientation, navigation, and communication. These abilities are crucial for their survival, allowing them to find food, mates, and suitable habitats while avoiding predators and navigating their environments effectively. Understanding these mechanisms provides insight into the complexity of animal behavior and the adaptations that have evolved over time.

Orientation

Orientation involves determining and maintaining a direction relative to an external reference. Animals use various cues for orientation, including the sun, stars, Earth's magnetic field, landmarks, and olfactory signals.

Sun Compass: Many animals, such as honeybees, use the sun as a compass. Honeybees, for instance, perform a "waggle dance" to communicate the direction and distance of food sources to their hive mates. This dance is oriented relative to the sun's position, which the bees can adjust for the time of day. Similarly, migratory birds like the European starling use the sun's position to navigate during their long migrations.

Magnetic Compass: The Earth's magnetic field is another crucial orientation cue. Birds like homing pigeons and European robins possess specialized magnetoreceptors that allow them to detect magnetic fields. These birds can use the Earth's magnetic field to determine their direction and navigate over long distances. Sea turtles also use magnetic fields to navigate across oceans, returning to the beaches where they were born to lay their eggs.

Star Compass: Night-migrating birds, such as the indigo bunting, use the stars to navigate. These birds have an innate ability to recognize constellations and use them to maintain a steady direction during their nocturnal migrations. Experiments have shown that young birds raised in a planetarium can learn to navigate using artificial star patterns, demonstrating the importance of stellar orientation.

Landmarks: Landmarks are physical features in the environment that animals use to orient themselves. Mammals like elephants and primates rely on landmarks for navigation. Elephants, known for their excellent memory, use landmarks such as rivers, mountains, and watering holes to navigate across vast distances. Similarly, chimpanzees use visual landmarks to find food sources and navigate their forest habitats.

Odor Cues: Olfactory cues play a significant role in the orientation of certain animals. Salmon, for example, use their keen sense of smell to locate their natal streams for spawning. These fish imprint on the unique chemical signature of their birthplace and can detect these odor cues even after several years in the ocean.

Navigation

Navigation is the process of determining and maintaining a course from one location to another. Animals employ various strategies for navigation, including piloting, path integration, celestial navigation, and the use of magnetic fields.

Piloting: Piloting involves using known landmarks to navigate. Dolphins, for instance, navigate using coastal landmarks and underwater features. They use their echolocation abilities to detect these landmarks and maintain a course. Piloting is also observed in terrestrial animals, such as wolves, which use familiar terrain features to navigate their territories.

Path Integration: Path integration, or dead reckoning, is a navigation strategy where animals keep track of the distance and direction travelled from a starting point. Ants, such as the desert ant Cataglyphis, are known for their remarkable path integration abilities. These ants can venture far from their nests in search of food and then return directly, even if they took a convoluted path to get there. They achieve this by continuously updating their position relative to their nest using visual cues and proprioceptive feedback.

Celestial Navigation: Celestial navigation involves using the sun, moon, and stars to navigate. Migratory birds are renowned for their ability to use celestial cues during their long-distance migrations. For instance, the Arctic tern travels from the Arctic to the Antarctic and back each year, navigating using a combination of the sun's position, the stars, and the Earth's magnetic field.

Use of Magnetic Fields: The Earth's magnetic field provides a reliable reference for navigation. Sea turtles are a prime example of animals using magnetic fields for navigation. Hatchlings, after emerging from their nests, quickly make their way to the ocean and embark on long migrations. They use the Earth's magnetic field to navigate across vast oceanic distances and return to the same beaches where they were born to lay their eggs as adults.

Communication

Communication is essential for social interactions, coordination, and survival in the animal kingdom. Animals use a variety of signals to communicate, including visual, auditory, chemical, tactile, and electrical signals.

Visual Signals: Visual signals are widely used in the animal kingdom for communication. Peacocks, for instance, use their elaborate plumage displays to attract mates. The vibrant colors and patterns of their feathers signal their health and genetic fitness to potential mates. Similarly, many species of birds use visual displays during courtship rituals to attract partners and establish territories.

Auditory Signals: Auditory signals, such as songs and calls, are crucial for communication in many animals. Birds are well-known for their complex songs, which serve various purposes, including attracting mates, defending territories, and coordinating group activities. For example, the songs of male songbirds are used to establish and defend territories during the breeding season. Dolphins also use a sophisticated system of vocalizations, including clicks and whistles, to communicate with each other and coordinate hunting activities.

Chemical Signals: Chemical signals, or pheromones, are widely used for communication, particularly among insects. Ants use pheromones to mark trails to food sources and signal alarm when a threat is detected. These chemical signals are highly specific and can convey detailed information about the nature and location of resources or dangers. Mammals also use chemical signals for communication. For instance, many mammals use scent marking to establish territories and convey information about their reproductive status.

Tactile Signals: Tactile communication involves physical contact between individuals. Primates, such as chimpanzees, use grooming as a form of tactile communication to strengthen social bonds and establish social hierarchies. Elephants use their trunks to touch and cares each other, reinforcing social bonds and providing comfort in stressful situations. Tactile communication is essential for maintaining social cohesion and coordination in many animal groups.

Electrical Signals: Electric fish, such as the electric eel, use electrical signals for communication and navigation. These fish generate electric fields and use them to detect objects in their environment and communicate with other electric fish. The electric signals can convey information about the sender's size, sex, and reproductive status. This form of communication is particularly useful in murky waters where visual signals are less effective.

Conclusion

Orientation, navigation, and communication are fundamental behaviours that animals have evolved to survive and reproduce. These behaviours are supported by a wide range of sensory and cognitive abilities, demonstrating the remarkable adaptability and intelligence of animals. From the use of the sun and stars for orientation to the sophisticated vocalizations and chemical signals used in communication, animals have developed diverse strategies to interact with their environments and each other. Understanding these behaviours provides valuable insights into the complexity of animal life and the evolutionary processes that shape these remarkable adaptations.

MCQ's

1. Which of the following mechanisms do birds primarily use to navigate during migration?
   - a) Solar navigation
   - b) Magnetic fields
   - c) Stellar navigation
   - d) All of the above
2. The waggle dance performed by honeybees is used to communicate information about:
   - a) The location of a new hive
   - b) The presence of predators
   - c) The direction and distance to a food source
   - d) The availability of water

3. Which of the following animals is known for its ability to use Earth's magnetic field for navigation?
   a) Monarch butterflies
   b) Pigeons
   c) Sea turtles
   d) All of the above
4. Bats use echolocation primarily to:
   a) Navigate in the dark
   b) Communicate with other bats
   c) Locate food
   d) Both a and c
5. Which sensory modality do salmon use to return to their natal streams for spawning?
   a) Visual cues
   b) Olfactory cues
   c) Magnetic fields
   d) Acoustic signals
6. In the context of animal communication, pheromones are:
   a) Visual signals
   b) Chemical signals
   c) Acoustic signals
   d) Tactile signals
7. Dolphins use which form of communication to identify each other?
   a) Visual signals
   b) Signature whistles
   c) Body language
   d) Tail slapping
8. What is the primary purpose of bird song?
   a) To navigate
   b) To attract mates and defend territory
   c) To warn of predators
   d) To communicate food locations
9. Which of the following animals is known for using complex vocalizations for communication within social groups?
   a) Wolves
   b) Elephants
   c) Dolphins
   d) All of the above
10. Fireflies use bioluminescence primarily for:
    a) Navigation
    b) Communication
    c) Predation
    d) Thermoregulation
11. Which animal is known for its remarkable ability to navigate using the stars?
    a) Monarch butterfly
    b) Desert ant
    c) Homing pigeon
    d) Dung beetle
12. What is the term for the phenomenon where animals return to their birthplace to reproduce?
    a) Homing
    b) Migration
    c) Natal philopatry
    d) Imprinting
13. Sea turtles use which cues to navigate to their nesting beaches?
    a) Magnetic fields
    b) Wave direction
    c) Chemical cues
    d) All of the above

14. Which type of navigation involves using the position of the sun?
   a) True navigation b) Compass orientation
   c) Path integration d) Dead reckoning
15. The ability of certain animals to orient themselves using the Earth's magnetic field is called:
   a) Phototaxis b) Chemotaxis
   c) Magnetoreception d) Thermoregulation
16. Which animal uses infrasound for long-distance communication?
   a) Dolphins b) Elephants
   c) Bats d) Whales
17. In which animal is the "dance language" used to communicate the location of resources?
   a) Ants b) Bees
   c) Termites d) Spiders
18. What is the primary purpose of alarm calls in many bird species?
   a) To attract mates b) To warn conspecifics of predators
   c) To establish territory d) To signal food presence
19. Which of the following animals uses a "foot drumming" behavior as a form of communication?
   a) Kangaroos b) Rabbits
   c) Elephants d) Beavers
20. Prairie dogs have a sophisticated communication system that can convey information about:
   a) The size and shape of a predator
   b) The speed of an approaching threat
   c) The type of predator
   d) All of the above
21. Which of the following animals uses the sun compass for navigation?
   a) Honeybees b) Sea turtles
   c) Monarch butterflies d) All of the above
22. What type of navigation involves calculating one's position based on a known starting point and using external cues?
   a) Compass orientation b) Path integration
   c) Landmark navigation d) Dead reckoning
23. Which of the following animals is known for its ability to perform long-distance migration using multiple cues, including magnetic fields and the position of the sun and stars?
   a) Salmon b) Monarch butterflies
   c) Arctic terns d) Homing pigeons

24. Which animal uses visual landmarks for navigation?
    a) Ants b) Bats
    c) Dolphins d) Whales
25. What is the primary method of navigation used by homing pigeons?
    a) Magnetic fields b) Olfactory cues
    c) Visual landmarks d) All of the above
26. Which type of communication is used by ants to lead other ants to a food source?
    a) Acoustic signals b) Visual signals
    c) Pheromonal trails d) Tactile signals
27. Which animal is known for using a complex system of vocalizations to communicate different types of information, such as identity and emotional state?
    a) Dolphins b) Lions
    c) Wolves d) Birds
28. Which of the following is an example of tactile communication?
    a) Elephants touching trunks
    b) Birds singing
    c) Bees performing the waggle dance
    d) Wolves howling
29. Which form of communication involves the use of body movements to convey messages?
    a) Acoustic signals b) Chemical signals
    c) Visual signals d) Tactile signals
30. Which bird species is famous for its incredible migratory journey from the Arctic to the Antarctic and back?
    a) Bald eagle b) Albatross
    c) Arctic tern d) Peregrine falcon
31. Which insect is known for its ability to navigate back to its hive after foraging over long distances?
    a) Butterfly b) Honeybee
    c) Dragonfly d) Moth
32. Which type of animal is known to use the angle of polarized light for navigation?
    a) Fish b) Birds
    c) Insects d) Mammals
33. Which marine animal is known to use echolocation for navigation and hunting?
    a) Sharks b) Whales
    c) Sea turtles d) Octopuses
34. Which of the following is a common form of communication among primates?
    a) Echolocation b) Pheromones
    c) Vocalizations and gestures d) Bioluminescence

35. Which animal uses tail slapping on the water surface as a warning signal to others?
    a) Dolphins
    b) Beavers
    c) Seals
    d) Otters
36. What is the primary form of communication used by wolves within their pack?
    a) Visual signals
    b) Vocalizations (howling)
    c) Chemical signals
    d) Tactile signals
37. Which type of communication involves the use of chemical substances released into the environment?
    a) Visual communication
    b) Tactile communication
    c) Acoustic communication
    d) Chemical communication
38. Which animal is known for using celestial navigation by observing the position of stars?
    a) Homing pigeon
    b) Desert ant
    c) European robin
    d) Dung beetle
39. Which type of navigation relies on the animal's internal sense of direction and distance travelled?
    a) Compass orientation
    b) Path integration
    c) True navigation
    d) Landmark navigation
40. Which animal uses chemical trails for orientation and navigation?
    a) Ants
    b) Birds
    c) Dolphins
    d) Bats
41. Which of the following animals is known to migrate vertically in the water column on a daily basis?
    a) Whales
    b) Sea turtles
    c) Zooplankton
    d) Sharks
42. Which mechanism do homing pigeons use as one of their primary means of navigation?
    a) Echolocation
    b) Magnetic field detection
    c) Infrared sensing
    d) UV light detection
43. Which type of communication is primarily used by frogs during the mating season?
    a) Chemical signals
    b) Visual signals
    c) Acoustic signals
    d) Tactile signals
44. Which animal is known for its ability to communicate through electric fields?
    a) Electric eel
    b) Platypus
    c) Star-nosed mole
    d) All of the above
45. What is the primary purpose of scent marking in many mammals?
    a) Navigation
    b) Foraging
    c) Territorial boundaries and social hierarchy
    d) Predation

46. Which type of animal is known to use bioluminescent signals for mating and attracting prey?
    a) Fireflies b) Anglerfish
    c) Jellyfish d) All of the above
47. Which animal is known for using the Earth's magnetic field to navigate over long distances?
    a) Monarch butterfly b) Loggerhead sea turtle
    c) Arctic tern d) Honeybee
48. What is the term for the ability of animals to find their way back to a specific location using environmental cues?
    a) Homing b) Migration
    c) Foraging d) Dispersal
49. Which bird is known to use infrasound to help navigate during migration?
    a) Homing pigeon b) Bar-tailed godwit
    c) Golden plover d) Swift
50. Which of the following is a method used by sea turtles to navigate the open ocean?
    a) Stellar navigation b) Scent trails
    c) Wave direction d) Electromagnetic reception
51. Which animal uses "dead reckoning" to navigate without external cues?
    a) Migratory birds b) Desert ants
    c) Salmon d) Elephants
52. Which animal uses ultrasonic calls for communication and navigation?
    a) Dogs b) Bats
    c) Elephants d) Dolphins
53. Which type of communication is commonly used by social insects like ants and bees?
    a) Visual signals b) Acoustic signals
    c) Chemical signals d) Tactile signals
54. In which species do males often use vocalizations to attract females during the mating season?
    a) Frogs b) Lions
    c) Butterflies d) Bees
55. Which form of communication involves the release and detection of airborne chemical signals?
    a) Visual communication b) Acoustic communication
    c) Pheromonal communication d) Tactile communication
56. Which insect uses the polarization pattern of the sky to navigate?
    a) Honeybee b) Dragonfly
    c) Butterfly d) Ant

57. Which animal is known for its ability to navigate using smell, specifically to find its breeding grounds?
    a) Monarch butterfly
    b) Salmon
    c) Sea turtle
    d) Bat
58. What is the main navigation tool used by nocturnal birds during migration?
    a) Magnetic fields
    b) Moonlight
    c) Stars
    d) Sunlight
59. Which of the following animals is known to use path integration for navigation?
    a) Elephants
    b) Bees
    c) Pigeons
    d) Desert ants
60. Which animal uses a combination of visual landmarks and magnetic fields to navigate?
    a) Dolphin
    b) Sea turtle
    c) Pigeon
    d) Whale
61. Which type of animal communication involves the use of body movements and visual signals?
    a) Acoustic communication
    b) Chemical communication
    c) Visual communication
    d) Tactile communication
62. Which type of animal is known to use color changes in their skin as a form of communication?
    a) Birds
    b) Fish
    c) Cephalopods (like octopuses and squids)
    d) Mammals
63. Which form of communication is primarily used by fireflies to attract mates?
    a) Acoustic signals
    b) Chemical signals
    c) Visual signals
    d) Tactile signals
64. Which of the following animals is known for its ability to navigate using the Earth's magnetic field?
    a) Dolphin
    b) Honeybee
    c) Salmon
    d) Monarch butterfly
65. What term describes the phenomenon where animals move from one region to another, typically on a seasonal basis?
    a) Hibernation
    b) Migration
    c) Estivation
    d) Territoriality
66. Which of the following is a primary method used by birds for long-distance migration?
    a) Sun compass
    b) Star compass
    c) Magnetic compass
    d) All of the above

67. Which of the following is NOT a method of animal navigation?
a) Path integration
b) Magnetic orientation
c) Echolocation
d) Photosynthesis

68. What is the primary function of the 'echolocation' used by bats and dolphins?
a) Finding mates
b) Locating prey
c) Marking territory
d) Communicating with conspecifics

69. Which animal is known for using a 'mental map' to navigate through complex environments?
a) Sea turtle
b) Homing pigeon
c) Squirrel
d) Wolf

70. The 'bee dance' includes which of the following types of movements to indicate distance and direction to a food source?
a) Circle dance
b) Waggle dance
c) Line dance
d) Spiral dance

71. What mechanism do sea turtles primarily use to return to their natal beaches for nesting?
a) Olfactory cues
b) Magnetic cues
c) Visual landmarks
d) Acoustic signals

Answer Key

1	d	2	c	3	d	4	d	5	b	6	b	7	b
8	b	9	d	10	b	11	d	12	c	13	d	14	b
15	c	16	b	17	b	18	b	19	a	20	d	21	d
22	d	23	c	24	a	25	d	26	c	27	a	28	b
29	c	30	c	31	b	32	c	33	b	34	c	35	b
36	b	37	d	38	d	39	b	40	a	41	c	42	b
43	c	44	a	45	c	46	d	47	b	48	a	49	a
50	c	51	b	52	b	53	c	54	a	55	c	56	a
57	b	58	c	59	d	60	c	61	c	62	c	63	c
64	d	65	b	66	d	67	d	68	b	69	b	70	b
71	b												

9

Overview of Cooperation and Kinship

Sourav Sikdar

Department of Zoology, Brahmananda Keshab Chandra College, Kolkata - 700 108, West Bengal

Introduction

Cooperation is an extensive wonder. Biologists refer this term communication as mutually advantageous interplays that occur with things of the unchanging species. Cooperation in animals performs to occur generally for direct benefit or middle from two points relatives. Spending opportunity and possessions helping a related individual grant permission initially appear destructive to an animal's chances of endurance but is actually advantageous over the enduring. However, few researchers, like Tim Clutton-Brock, assert that communication service is a more intricate process. They state that helpers can sustain more direct, and less unintended, gains from assisting possible choice than it is usually stated. These gains include guardianship from predatoriness and increased generative appropriateness. Furthermore, they claim that cooperation concede possibility not only be an interplay between two things but can be part of the more extensive aim of uniting populations. A generalized birth of progress that normalizes competition as a big method casts unity as a paradox, faraway in a confuse place survival is calculated in agreements of costs and benefits, following the market rule of self-addition. Prominent biologists, such as Charles Darwin, E. O. Wilson, and W. D. Hamilton, have erect the development of cooperation spellbinding because evolutionary theory favors those who attain prominent supporter generative success while joint attitude often decreases the generative benefit of the player (the individual performing the helpful attitude).

Hence, participation seemed to pose a question to the theory of evolutionary theory, that rests provided that individuals spar to recover and be dramatic their reproductive accomplishments. Additionally, few species have happened raise to act cooperative presence that grant permission on the face of it seem damaging to their own developmental fitness. For example, when a ground hoard sounds an alarm welcome caution other group appendage of a nearby dog, it draws consideration to itself and increases allure own advantage of being eaten. There have happened diversified theories for the evolution of assistance, all of that are implanted in Hamilton's models based on all-embracing appropriateness. These models hypothesize that unity is popular by evolutionary theory due to either direct appropriateness benefits (together advantageous cooperation) or roundabout appropriateness benefits (altruistic partnership).

Kinship or Kin selection may define as a form of 'helping behaviour' of animals favoured by Natural Selection through the benefit obtained by genetically related individuals, the relatives or Kin, in the form of increased survival value and reproductive success. The principle of kinship is that- "the decrease in an individual's fitness as a result of its spending time and energy helping it's relatives (Kins) is more than compensated for by the increased fitness of its relatives (Kins)". This, therefore, contrasts with the selection confined solely to an individual and its own offspring. On the other hand, altruism is the act at which point the player (individual that completes activity the operation) pays appropriateness cost to the receiver that gets the benefit.

MCQ's

1. Which of the following is not a theory that describes, explains, or predicts what motivates helping behavior?
   a) Reciprocal innervation. b) Social norms.
   c) Evolutionary theory. d) The social exchange theory
2. The idea of kin selection is used to describe and predict _______________.
   a) When people help other people
   b) Why people help other people
   c) Who will help another person
   d) How to increase helping another person
3. The term egoism refers to
   a) Arrogance
   b) Someone who is overconfident.
   c) The idea that people do what is best for themselves.
   d) A person who is "full of themselves."
4. Altruism is
   a) A belief in all things that are true.
   b) Doing something good for one's self.
   c) Doing something neutral for others.
   d) Doing something good for others without expecting anything in return.
5. Research has shown that increasing a person's self-awareness _____________ helping behavior.
   a) Decreases b) Increases
   c) Has no effect on d) Has a negative effect on
6. Jerry borrows a power saw from Joe, who lives next door. A week later, when Joe's lawn mower breaks, Joe borrows Jerry's lawn mower. This exemplifies
   a) Social exchange theory b) Reciprocal disinhibition
   c) The reciprocity norm d) Social capital
7. Which country is more likely to support the social responsibility norm?
   a) United States b) Europe
   c) Canada d) India

8. People will become organ donors to those outside of their families, in part, because of the
   a) Social responsibility norm
   b) Social exchange theory
   c) The reciprocity norm
   d) Kin selection theory
9. One way to increase helping behavior is
   a) To decrease empathy
   b) To model altruism
   c) To remove people's guilt
   d) To increase the number of bystanders
10. If an ambiguous situation is made clear, this will ______________ helping behavior
   a) Increase
   b) Decrease
   c) Not have an effect on
   d) Have the reverse effect on
11. Bystander inaction increases
   a) As the bystanders become more leisurely.
   b) As the bystanders are more observant.
   c) As the number of bystanders increases.
   d) As the number of bystanders decreases.
12. Research has shown that if people are made to feel guilty, this will __________ helping behavior.
   a) Increase
   b) Decrease
   c) Have no effect on
   d) Have a detrimental effect on
13. Responsibility diffusion
   a) Increases helpfulness.
   b) Has no effect on helping behavior.
   c) Can lead to more helping behavior.
   d) Can lead to less helping behavior.
14. Regarding the idea of kin selection, who is most likely to receive help first?
   a) A stranger before a family member.
   b) A stranger before a neighbor.
   c) A grandparent before a child.
   d) A child before a grandparent.
15. When people show a lack of inclusion in their circle of moral concern, this is referred to as
   a) Moral exclusion.
   b) Ostracism.
   c) Saving social capital.
   d) The overjustification effect.
16. What role does similarity play in helping behavior?
   a) The more dissimilar a person is to a potential helper, the more the potential helper will offer to help.
   b) The more similar a person is to a potential helper, the more the potential helper will offer to help.
   c) The more similar a person is to a potential helper, the less the potential helper will offer to help.
   d) The more similar a person is to a potential helper, the more the potential helper will ignore the person in need.

17. Before agreeing to help out at the homeless shelter, Sharon weighs the costs (e.g., getting up at dawn on a Saturday) and benefits (e.g., feeling good about helping others) of doing so. This strategy would be predicted by

    a) The empathy/altruism hypothesis. b) Social exchange theory.

    c) The social responsibility norm. d) Social comparison theory.

18. When it is close to the holidays, we all often receive many free gifts from charity groups and churches. Generally, after receiving this small token, we feel obligated to make a donation. This best illustrates

    a) The social exchange theory. b) Egoism.

    c) The reciprocity norm. d) Social capital.

19. Which technique has been used in research to elicit helping behavior?

    a) The door-in-the-face technique.

    b) The foot-in-the-mouth technique.

    c) The toe-in-the-door technique

    d) The door-behind-the-screen technique.

20. Reciprocity among humans is

    a) Stronger in rural villages than in big cities.

    b) Stronger in big cities than in rural villages.

    c) Rarely seen in individualistic societies.

    d) Rarely seen in collectivistic societies.

21. Which of these is a form of kin selection?

    a) A squirrel screeching out an alarm call when a dangerous bird is nearby. The alarm will get the bird's attention, and the squirrel giving the warning might die, but other squirrels nearby will have the chance to get to safety.

    b) A cat hunting small birds and animals to get enough protein to nourish her growing kittens

    c) A wasp laying its eggs inside a living caterpillar. The caterpillar will die as the hatched wasps feed on its tissue.

    d) Bears hibernating for the winter. If they did not eat enough during the summer and fall months, they will not have enough stored energy to make it through the non-feeding times.

22. Kin selection theory explains which of these strange insects?

    a) Wasps that parasitize living things

    b) Cicadas that live underground for 17 years

    c) Termite colonies that are mostly sterile females with one fertile queen

    d) Cockroaches that live in large colonies

23. What is altruism?

    a) When an individual causes harm to another for the benefit of the individual

    b) When two individuals work together for the mutual benefit of both

    c) When two individuals interact with no benefit for either of them

    d) When an individual causes self harm for the good of another; selfless behavior

24. Arguments that a particular behavior has been selected for because it benefits the population or species are examples of arguments for
    a) Kin selection b) Sexual selection
    c) Group selection d) Natural selection
25. What type of selection is most likely responsible for the large antlers seen on male elk?
    a) Kin selection b) Group selection
    c) Territorial selection d) Intrasexual selection
26. Which of the following Belding's ground squirrels is most likely to give an alarm call?
    a) A female with no kin nearby b) A female with kin nearby
    c) A male with no kin nearby d) A male with kin nearby
27. Selection that favors altruism for the propagation of alleles in a "family" is called kin selection.
    a) True b) False
    c) Both d) None
28. Some male birds that did not find a mate will help raise the offspring of a relative. This self-sacrifice is best known as:
    a) Altruistic behavior b) Selfish behavior
    c) Cooperative behavior d) Spiteful behavior
29. Which of the following is commonly identified as a risk to living in a social group?
    a) Increase in the spread of diseases
    b) Decrease in competition for mates
    c) Decrease in protection from predators
    d) Increase in available food
30. Learning is change in behaviour as a result of
    a) Imprinting b) Altruism
    c) Instinct d) Experience
31. A process in which an animal sacrifices its reproductive potential for the benefit of another organism is called
    a) Mutualism b) Cooperation
    c) Altruism d) Autism
32. The behaviour in which one animal is aggressive or attacks another animal, the other responds by returning the aggression or submitting is called:
    a) Agnostic b) Territory
    c) Hierarchy d) Altruism
33. Which of the following is not an intra-specific relationship?
    a) Territoriality b) Competition
    c) Cooperation d) Symbiosis

34. Which of the following statements is true?
    a) Cooperation is based on emotional relationship, harmony and intimacy
    b) Accommodation is the situation of tolerating one another without interference.
    c) Both a and b are correct
    d) Both a and b are false
35. A social position has two parts. They are
    a) Obligations and rights b) Rights and conflicts
    c) Cooperation and conflict d) Rights and statuses
36. The prevalence of village exogamy in North India arises from which of the following highly interrelated factors?
    1. Caste endogamy
    2. Local fictive kinship
    3. Territorial stabilization of kin groups
    4. Gotra

    Select the correct answer using the code given below:
    a) 1 and 3 only b) 1, 2 and 4 only
    c) 2 and 4 only d) 1, 2, 3 and 4
37. Behaviour that is valued by others in a particular culture is known as ______
    a) Prosocial behaviour b) Helping behaviour
    c) Altruism d) None of these
38. Helping behaviour includes-
    a) Includes actions that only benefit the self
    b) Includes actions that benefit others and the self in the same instance
    c) Is defined as behaviour that only benefits others and does not benefit the self
    d) None of these
39. The ability of kin to survive and reproduce is known as __________.
    a) Natural selection b) Altruistic behavior
    c) Inclusive fitness d) Selfish behavior
40. Male baboons establish higher or lower rankings among themselves through confrontations; this determines their _______.
    a) Imprinting level b) Fixed action pattern
    c) Territoriality d) Altruism
41. When a red deer stag or male songbird defends a certain area, he is showing ________.
    a) Imprinting level b) Fixed action pattern
    c) Territoriality d) Altruism

42. Evolution by ________ can occur when females have the opportunity to select among potential mates and or when males compete among themselves for access to reproductive females.
   a) Imprinting
   b) Sexual selection
   c) Sociality
   d) Altruism
   e) Dominance hierarchy
43. ______ applies the principles of evolutionary biology to the study of social behavior in animals.
   a) Altruism
   b) Behaviorism
   c) Genetics
   d) Sociobiology
44. Altruism is behavior performed for selfish survival of one individual.
   a) True
   b) False
45. The theory of inclusive fitness predicts that __________.
   a) There is no value to passing on your own genes by reproducing yourself
   b) Helping any member of your species is of value to passing on your own genes
   c) Helping close relatives reproduce will ensure your genes are passed on even if you never reproduce.
   d) The more advanced the animal, the more likely it will be altruistic
   e) All behavior is altruistic
46. Kin selection is favoured by-
   a) Genetic drift
   b) Natural Selection
   c) Natural calamities
   d) Adaptive radiation
47. Kin selection increase its relatives'
   a) Fitness
   b) Fecundity rate
   c) Breeding capacity
   d) Feeding behavior
48. Social insects select the following option in relation to kin selection-
   a) Females produce her own offspring only
   b) Help the colony to produce reproductives
   c) Both a & b
   d) None of the above
49. 'Full sibs' mean-
   a) If the father of the reproductives is her own father
   b) If the reproductives are fathered by a different male
   c) Both a & b
   d) None of the above
50. 'Half sibs' mean-
   a) If the father of the reproductives is her own father
   b) If the reproductives are fathered by a different male
   c) Both a & b
   d) None of the above

51. In the social insect colony, Queen is-
 a) Not protected b) Protected
 c) Protect others d) No event about protection
52. Who from the followings didn't show Kin selection
 a) Saturniid Moths in Barro Colorado Island
 b) Wasps
 c) Bees
 d) Bats
53. Who from the followings is reputed for Kin selection studies?
 a) Thompson b) Blest
 c) Taylor d) Crick
54. Kin selection is important for a species population at the cost of-
 a) A group of members b) An individual member
 c) The relatives d) Queen
55. First scientist to give the mathematical module of kin selection is-
 a) Andre Adams b) Hamilton
 c) Kevin d) Blest
56. Reciprocal altruism means-
 a) One reciprocates other b) One helps and other benefited
 c) One survives and other dead d) No one help others
57. Vampire bats show-
 a) Altruism b) Kinship
 c) Reciprocal altruism d) Parasitism
58. Kin selection does not involve-
 a) Helping behavior b) Caring
 c) Feeding d) Reciprocation
59. Reciprocal altruism applied for who have-
 a) Capacity to help b) Capacity to fed
 c) Good memories d) Better strength
60. Individuals can recognize each other in case of-
 a) Altruistic behaviour b) Reciprocal altruism
 c) Learning behaviour d) Selfishness
61. The theory of reciprocal altruism in Vampire bat was proposed by-
 a) Taylor b) Wilkinson
 c) Fransis d) Rafael
62. Reciprocal Altruism is advantageous to increase-
 a) Survival chance b) Death rate
 c) Food searching d) All of the above

63. Cooperation is a type of
    a) Genetical behaviour
    b) Social behavior
    c) Physiological behavior
    d) Anatomical behavior
64. Animal cooperation is-
    a) Mutually beneficial
    b) Not beneficial
    c) One sided benefit
    d) None of the above
65. During prey hunting, chimpanzees produce a
    a) "Normal bark"
    b) "Hunting bark"
    c) "Shouting only"
    d) "Making signal"
66. Ants might work together to carry a large insect back to the nest in order to feed other ants is an example of-
    a) Selfishness
    b) Animal cooperation
    c) Reproductive behavior
    d) All of the above
67. The ability to reproduce is greatly enhanced through
    a) Reproductive behavior
    b) Animal cooperation
    c) Selfishness
    d) All of the above
68. Collaboration is most common among individuals with
    a) Similar genetic backgrounds
    b) Different genetic background
    c) Genetic background not required
    d) None of the above
69. Social structures and cooperation may be strengthened by-
    a) Connecting among same individuals
    b) Make a proper community
    c) Making self-reinforcing feedback loop
    d) All of the above
70. Which one of the following is a type of social behavior observed in animals that is mutually beneficial?
    a) Cooperation
    b) Selfishness
    c) Spitefulness
    d) None of the above
71. Cooperative behavior can be
    a) Either mutualistic or altruistic
    b) Mutualistic
    c) Altruistic
    d) both mutualistic & altruistic
72. Reduce their own offspring production but boost the number of offspring that other animals might produce is called-
    a) Cooperative behavior
    b) Mutualism
    c) Commensalism
    d) Parasitism
73. In the presence of a predator, Vervet monkey (*Chlorocebus pygerythrus*) emit warning calls to warn other monkeys. As a result, they attract the predator's attention. It's an example of-
    a) Altruism
    b) Mutualism
    c) Commensalism
    d) Parasitism

74. Among many types of cooperative behavior, there are three that are especially common-
   a) Mutualism, group hunting & group seeking
   b) Cooperative group hunting, Cooperative safekeeping & Cooperative territory protection (scent marking, howling)
   c) Group calling, group hunting & group seeking
   d) None of the above

75. During hunting, bottlenose dolphins form groups of
   a) 5-6 dolphins b) 10 dolphins
   c) 8-10 dolphins d) More than 10 dolphins

76. Sometimes cooperative hunting is seen
   a) Among many species b) Among 3 species
   c) Between two different species. d) None of the above

77. Some animals can exhibit cooperative behavior as a means of
   a) Safekeeping and defense. b) Self-protection
   c) Self-survival d) None of the above

78. Cooperative territory protection found in -
   a) Wolves b) Buffalo
   c) Cow d) Deer

79. Lions cooperate to hunt, defend territory, raise young, repel male challengers, and more is the unique example of-
   a) Cooperation b) Mutualism
   c) Commensalism d) Parasitism

80. During cooperative prey capture, how many spiders are needed to capture large prey?
   a) 20 b) 30
   c) 25 d) 50

81. What are the common examples of cooperation?
   a) Group hunting, babysitting, utilizing sentries, or fighting as a group.
   b) Territory marking
   c) Hunting and nesting
   d) None of the above

82. Who might be the most cooperative, sharing responsibility in nearly all aspects of their lives?
   a) Deers b) Meerkats
   c) Tigers d) Ants

83. Which one from the followings is NOT the common type of signal for communication?
   a) Pheromones b) Auditory cues
   c) Chasing d) Visual cues

84. A pheromone is a type of
   a) Chemical signal   b) Physical signal
   c) Tactile signal   d) Visual signal
85. Auditory communication is particularly important in
   a) Dogs   b) Birds
   c) Dolphins   d) Wasps
86. Facial expressions is a type of-
   a) Chemical signal   b) Physical signal
   c) Tactile signal   d) Visual signal
87. Tactile signal means-
   a) Speech   b) Touch
   c) vision   d) None of the above
88. Cooperation in animals appears to occur mostly for
   a) Help others
   b) Direct benefit or between relatives.
   c) Social communication
   d) None of these
89. What is the main purpose of cooperation?
   a) To provide goods and services.   b) To kill other relatives
   c) Complete dependency   d) All of the above
90. Which animal of the following show 'teamwork'?
   a) Wasps   b) Deer
   c) Humming bird   d) Bees
91. Which animals of the followings are selfless?
   a) Whales   b) Giraffe
   c) Donkey   d) Sunbird
92. The elements of kin selection lead directly to the concept now known as
   a) Chargaff's rule   b) Hamilton's rule
   c) Mangold's rule   d) None of the above
93. Who suggest the term 'mutual benefit' for behaviours that benefit both self and other?
   a) Hamilton   b) West et al.
   c) Mangold   d) None of the above
94. The theory of reciprocal altruism was originally developed by
   a) Trivers   b) Hamilton
   c) West   d) Mangold
95. Kin selection cannot help to explain altruism among
   a) Relatives   b) Neighbours
   c) Non-relatives   d) All of the above

96. Animal cooperation is explained by the theory of
    a) 'Goodness fit' b) 'Inclusive fitness'
    c) Hamilton's rule theory d) Game theory
97. The relationship between two animals called-
    a) Symbiosis b) Mutualism
    c) Commensalism d) Parasitism
98. Lions live in groups called
    a) Herd b) Batch
    c) Prides d) All of the above
99. Which animal from the following represents cooperation?
    a) Cow b) Cape buffalos
    c) Dog d) Cat
100. Which of the following is the symbol of peaceful animal?
    a) Cow b) Dove
    c) Dog d) Cat
101. Why do animals work together?
    a) For feeding b) For survival
    c) For reproduction d) For prey capturing
102. Electrical discharge is also an example of-
    a) Animal communication b) Kinship
    c) Commensalism d) Altruism
103. An animal that provides a signal is called
    a) A sender b) A receiver
    c) Vector d) All of the above
104. The animal to which the signal is directed is
    a) A sender b) The receiver
    c) Vector d) All of the above
105. The lowest frequencies of sound produced by-
    a) Birds b) Insects
    c) Mammals d) Annelids
106. Stridulation is the mechanism of sound production in certain species of
    a) Orthoptera b) Lepidoptera
    c) Hymenoptera d) Diptera
107. Vibrations is another type of
    a) Chemical signal b) Physical signal
    c) Tactile signal d) None of the above

108. Propagation of sound is complicated when
  a) The sender and receiver are in certain distance
  b) The sender and receiver are very close
  c) The sender and receiver are close to a boundary
  d) All of the above
109. Cephalopods do their communication by using their
  a) Eyes
  b) Adjustable lenses
  c) Tentacles
  d) Suckers
110. Which protein pigment is involved in colour absorption in multicellular organisms?
  a) Melanin
  b) Rhodopsin
  c) Keratin
  d) All of the above
111. Courtship signals are typically given by
  a) Females
  b) Males
  c) Both
  d) None

Answer Key

1	a	2	b	3	c	4	d	5	b	6	c	7	d
8	a	9	b	10	a	11	c	12	a	13	d	14	d
15	a	16	b	17	b	18	c	19	a	20	a	21	a
22	c	23	d	24	a	25	d	26	b	27	a	28	a
29	a	30	d	31	c	32	a	33	d	34	c	35	a
36	c	37	a	38	b	39	a	40	a	41	d	42	b
43	d	44	a	45	b	46	b	47	a	48	c	49	a
50	b	51	b	52	a	53	b	54	b	55	b	56	a
57	c	58	d	59	c	60	b	61	b	62	a	63	b
64	a	65	b	66	b	67	b	68	a	69	c	70	a
71	a	72	a	73	a	74	b	75	a	76	c	77	a
78	a	79	a	80	c	81	a	82	b	83	c	84	a
85	b	86	d	87	b	88	b	89	a	90	d	91	a
92	b	93	b	94	a	95	c	96		97	a	98	c
99	b	100	b	101	b	102	a	103	a	104	b	105	b
106	a	107	c	108	c	109	b	110	b	111	b		

10

Role of Hormones and Drugs on Animal Behaviour

Vandana Singh

Assistant Professor, Department of Veterinary Pharmacology and Toxicology, College of Veterinary and Animal Sciences, Kishanganj-Bihar – 855 107

Introduction

Animal behavior, a fascinating field of study, encompasses a wide range of activities and responses to internal and external stimuli. Among the various factors that shape these behaviour's, hormones and drugs are particularly significant. These biochemical agents profoundly influence the physiological and psychological aspects of animals, leading to observable changes in their behaviour. This introduction explores the roles of hormones and drugs in animal behavior, detailing their mechanisms, effects, and implications for broader scientific understanding and practical applications. Hormones and drugs play vital roles in shaping animal behavior through complex biochemical pathways. Hormones act as internal regulators, orchestrating responses to environmental and physiological changes, while drugs, whether therapeutic or environmental, modulate these processes, often with profound behavioral consequences. Understanding these influences is crucial for advancing animal welfare, conservation efforts, and biomedical research, ultimately enriching our comprehension of the intricate relationship between biology and behavior in the animal kingdom.

Hormones and Animal Behaviour Deliver

Hormones are chemical messengers produced by endocrine glands and secreted into the bloodstream, where they travel to target organs and tissues, eliciting specific physiological responses. These responses, in turn, influence behaviour. The following are some key hormones that play critical roles in animal behavior:

1. Corticosteroids

- **Function**: Corticosteroids, such as cortisol in mammals and corticosterone in birds and reptiles, are released by the adrenal glands in response to stress.
- **Behavioral Impact**: They prepare the body for the fight-or-flight response, affecting behaviour's related to fear, anxiety, and aggression. Chronic stress exposure and elevated corticosteroid levels can lead to long-term behavioral changes, including heightened anxiety and altered social interactions.

2. Sex Hormones

- **Testosterone**: This hormone, predominant in males, influences aggressive behavior, territoriality, and mating practices. For instance, higher testosterone levels are associated with increased aggression and dominance in many animal species.
- **Estrogen and Progesterone**: Predominant in females, these hormones regulate reproductive behaviours, maternal instincts, and mating receptivity. Estrogen, in particular, can enhance sexual attraction and readiness for mating.

3. Oxytocin and Vasopressin

- **Oxytocin**: Known as the "love hormone," oxytocin facilitates social bonding, parental care, and mating behaviours. It enhances trust and reduces fear responses in social contexts.
- **Vasopressin**: Similar to oxytocin, vasopressin influences social behaviours, including aggression and territoriality, particularly in males. It plays a role in pair-bond formation in some species.

4. Melatonin

- **Function**: Produced by the pineal gland, melatonin regulates circadian rhythms and seasonal behaviours.
- **Behavioral Impact**: It influences sleep-wake cycles, reproductive timing, and migration patterns. Changes in melatonin levels can affect seasonal breeding behaviours and photoperiodic responses.

5. Thyroid Hormones

- **Function**: Thyroid hormones, such as thyroxine (T4) and triiodothyronine (T3), regulate metabolism and energy levels.
- **Behavioral Impact**: They influence overall activity levels, mood, and cognitive functions. Hypothyroidism or hyperthyroidism can lead to lethargy, depression, or hyperactivity and anxiety, respectively.

Drugs and Animal Behavior-

Drugs, including those administered for medical purposes and those encountered in the environment, can significantly alter animal behavior. These substances can be broadly categorized based on their effects:

1. Psychoactive Drugs:

- **Antidepressants (e.g., SSRIs)**: Used to manage anxiety, depression, and compulsive behaviours in animals. They work by increasing serotonin levels in the brain, leading to mood stabilization and reduced anxiety.
- **Antipsychotics and Anxiolytics**: These drugs can calm aggressive animals, reduce fear, and manage behavioral disorders.

2. Narcotics and Stimulants

- **Opioids**: Used for pain management, these drugs can also induce euphoria or sedation, altering normal behaviours.

- **Amphetamines**: Stimulants that increase alertness, energy, and activity levels. They can lead to hyperactivity and increased risk-taking behaviours.

3. Environmental Contaminants

- **Pesticides and Heavy Metals**: Exposure to environmental pollutants can disrupt the nervous system and behavior. For example, pesticides have been shown to impair the foraging behavior of bees, which impacts pollination and ecological balance.
- **Endocrine Disruptors**: Chemicals that interfere with hormone function, leading to reproductive issues, altered growth patterns, and changes in social behaviours.

4. Recreational and Natural Psychoactive Substances

- **Fermented Fruits**: Some animals consume naturally occurring psychoactive substances, leading to behaviours akin to intoxication. This can affect their social interactions and risk-taking behaviours.
- **Cannabinoids and Hallucinogens**: Found in certain plants, these substances can alter perception, mood, and behavior in animals that ingest them.

Drugs influence animal behavior primarily through their actions on the central nervous system. They can alter neurotransmitter levels, receptor sensitivity, and neural circuitry, leading to changes in mood, cognition, and motor functions. The effects can be immediate, such as sedation or stimulation, or long-term, potentially causing dependency or chronic behavioral changes.

Implications and Applications

Understanding the role of hormones and drugs in animal behavior has significant implications for various fields:

1. Conservation Biology

- **Stress Responses**: Knowledge of how stress hormones affect behavior can help in developing strategies to reduce stress in captive and wild animals, improving their welfare and survival rates.
- **Pollution Impact**: Understanding the behavioral effects of environmental contaminants aids in assessing the ecological impact of pollution and developing conservation policies.

2. Animal Welfare and Veterinary Medicine

- **Behavioral Treatments**: Hormones and psychoactive drugs are used to manage behavioral disorders in domestic animals, improving their quality of life and human-animal interactions.
- **Pain Management**: Effective use of narcotics and other pain-relieving drugs ensures better management of pain in animals, reducing suffering and enhancing recovery.

3. Biomedical Research

- **Human Health Models**: Studying hormone and drug effects on animal behavior provides valuable insights into human psychiatric and neurological disorders. Animal models are crucial for developing and testing new treatments.

- **Pharmacology**: Research on how drugs affect animal behavior helps in understanding their mechanisms of action, side effects, and therapeutic potential.

4. Ethology and Neuroscience

- **Behavioral Ecology**: Insights into how hormones regulate behaviors like mating, aggression, and social bonding contribute to our understanding of animal ecology and evolution.
- **Neural Mechanisms**: Exploring how drugs influence neural activity and behavior enhances our knowledge of brain function and its relationship to behavior.

MCQ's

1. Which hormone is primarily involved in the regulation of aggressive behavior in many animals?
   a) Estrogen b) Oxytocin
   c) Testosterone d) Insulin
2. Which neurotransmitter is commonly associated with the regulation of mood and anxiety in animals?
   a) Dopamine b) Serotonin
   c) Acetylcholine d) Norepinephrine
3. What is the primary effect of the hormone oxytocin on social behavior in animals?
   a) Increases aggression
   b) Enhances maternal bonding and social interactions
   c) Reduces pain perception
   d) Stimulates appetite
4. Which class of drugs is often used to modify aggressive behavior in animals?
   a) Stimulants b) Antidepressants
   c) Benzodiazepines d) Antipsychotics
5. How does the hormone cortisol affect animal behavior during stressful situations?
   a) Reduces anxiety
   b) Increases social bonding
   c) Increases alertness and prepares for fight or flight
   d) Induces sleep
6. Which drug is commonly used in veterinary medicine to manage anxiety in animals?
   a) Diazepam b) Aspirin
   c) Ibuprofen d) Metformin
7. Which hormone is known to influence seasonal breeding patterns in many animals?
   a) Melatonin b) Prolactin
   c) Insulin d) Glucagon

8. What is the primary action of benzodiazepines in the treatment of animal behavior disorders?
   a) Increase the reuptake of serotonin
   b) Block the reuptake of dopamine
   c) Enhance the effect of the neurotransmitter GABA
   d) Increase the production of acetylcholine
9. Which hormone is primarily involved in the regulation of growth and development in young animals?
   a) Thyroxine b) Growth hormone
   c) Adrenaline d) Estrogen
10. Which hormone is responsible for regulating water balance and can affect animal behavior related to hydration?
   a) Oxytocin b) Antidiuretic hormone (ADH)
   c) Progesterone d) Cortisol
11. Which of the following is a common effect of sedative drugs on animal behavior?
   a) Increased aggression b) Hyperactivity
   c) Reduced anxiety and sedation d) Enhanced memory
12. What effect do stimulant drugs like amphetamines have on animals?
   a) Induce sleep
   b) Increase alertness and physical activity
   c) Decrease appetite
   d) Reduce anxiety
13. Which drug is often used to manage pain and can alter animal behavior by causing euphoria or sedation?
   a) Antibiotics b) Opioids
   c) Antifungals d) Antihistamines
14. How do antipsychotic drugs typically affect animal behavior?
   a) Increase aggressive behavior
   b) Reduce psychotic symptoms and may induce calmness
   c) Stimulate appetite
   d) Enhance motor coordination
15. What is a common behavioral effect of benzodiazepines in animals?
   a) Increase aggression
   b) Reduce anxiety and induce muscle relaxation
   c) Increase appetite
   d) Enhance memory retention
16. Which of the following drugs is used to treat anxiety and phobias in animals and is known to have a calming effect?
   a) Diazepam b) Aspirin
   c) Metformin d) Ibuprofen

17. How can chronic use of corticosteroids affect animal behavior?
    a) Induce sleep
    b) Cause hyperactivity and irritability
    c) Reduce aggression
    d) Increase social bonding
18. Which drug class is commonly used to treat depression in animals, potentially improving their overall mood and behavior?
    a) Stimulants b) Antidepressants
    c) Antihistamines d) Antibiotics
19. How do opioids affect animal behavior besides pain relief?
    a) Increase aggression b) Cause euphoria and sedation
    c) Enhance memory d) Increase alertness
20. What is a potential side effect of using anticholinergic drugs on animal behavior?
    a) Increased salivation b) Enhanced memory
    c) Confusion and disorientation d) Reduced aggression
21. Which hormone is primarily responsible for the "fight or flight" response?
    a) Estrogen b) Insulin
    c) Cortisol d) Melatonin
22. Which neurotransmitter is commonly associated with pleasure and reward in the brain?
    a) Dopamine b) Serotonin
    c) Acetylcholine d) GABA
23. What is the main effect of the hormone oxytocin on human behavior?
    a) Increases aggression
    b) Enhances social bonding and trust
    c) Reduces pain perception
    d) Stimulates hunger
24. Which class of drugs is typically used to treat anxiety disorders?
    a) Stimulants b) Opioids
    c) Benzodiazepines d) Antipsychotics
25. What effect does the hormone melatonin have on the body?
    a) Regulates sleep-wake cycles b) Increases alertness
    c) Stimulates muscle growth d) Controls appetite
26. Which drug is commonly used to manage symptoms of depression?
    a) Aspirin b) Sertraline
    c) Diazepam d) Methamphetamine
27. Which hormone is known as the "stress hormone"?
    a) Thyroxine b) Cortisol
    c) Testosterone d) Progesterone

28. What is the primary action of antidepressants known as selective serotonin reuptake inhibitors (SSRIs)?
    a) Increase the reuptake of serotonin
    b) Block the reuptake of serotonin
    c) Increase the production of dopamine
    d) Block the reuptake of dopamine
29. Which neurotransmitter imbalance is most commonly associated with Parkinson's disease?
    a) Excess serotonin
    b) Low levels of dopamine
    c) High levels of acetylcholine
    d) Low levels of GABA
30. Which hormone is primarily involved in regulating metabolism?
    a) Growth hormone
    b) Insulin
    c) Thyroid hormone
    d) Adrenaline

Hormones and Animal Behavior

1. Which hormone is known as the "stress hormone" in humans?
    a) Testosterone
    b) Estrogen
    c) Cortisol
    d) Insulin
2. What effect does high testosterone have on male animal behavior?
    a) Increased nurturing behavior
    b) Decreased aggression
    c) Increased aggression
    d) Decreased sexual activity
3. Which hormone is primarily responsible for regulating sleep-wake cycles?
    a) Oxytocin
    b) Melatonin
    c) Prolactin
    d) Adrenaline
4. Prolactin is crucial for which type of behavior in mammals?
    a) Aggression
    b) Parental care
    c) Mating
    d) Feeding
5. Oxytocin is often referred to as what?
    a) The stress hormone
    b) The hunger hormone
    c) The love hormone
    d) The sleep hormone
6. Which hormone increases appetite and food-seeking behavior?
    a) Leptin
    b) Insulin
    c) Ghrelin
    d) Estrogen
7. What effect does high levels of estrogen have on female animal behavior?
    a) Increased aggression
    b) Decreased mating behavior
    c) Increased receptivity to mating
    d) Decreased nurturing behavior
8. Which hormone is produced in response to darkness and helps regulate circadian rhythms?
    a) Melatonin
    b) Cortisol
    c) Prolactin
    d) Oxytocin

9. What is the primary function of leptin in regulating animal behavior?
   a) Stimulating appetite
   b) Increasing aggression
   c) Promoting satiety and reducing food intake
   d) Enhancing mating behavior
10. Elevated levels of which hormone are linked to maternal behaviors in many species?
   a) Testosterone b) Progesterone
   c) Cortisol d) Insulin

Drugs and Animal Behavior

11. Which drug is commonly used to treat anxiety and affects serotonin levels?
   a) Caffeine b) Prozac (Fluoxetine)
   c) Nicotine d) Alcohol
12. What effect does caffeine have on animal behavior?
   a) Decreases alertness
   b) Increases aggression
   c) Enhances alertness and reduces fatigue
   d) Promotes sleep
13. Which drug is known for its calming effects and is often used to treat anxiety?
   a) Amphetamine b) Diazepam (Valium)
   c) Cocaine d) Nicotine
14. What behavioral effect does nicotine have on animals?
   a) Increases appetite
   b) Decreases aggression
   c) Stimulates alertness and reduces anxiety
   d) Induces sleep
15. Alcohol has what kind of effect on animal behavior?
   a) Stimulant b) Depressant
   c) Hallucinogenic d) No effect
16. Amphetamines are known to have which effect on animal behavior?
   a) Increase appetite b) Decrease aggression
   c) Increase activity and alertness d) Promote sleep
17. Which drug is commonly used to induce sleep in animals?
   a) Caffeine b) Morphine
   c) Melatonin d) Nicotine
18. Morphine is used for what primary effect on animal behavior?
   a) Pain relief and sedation b) Increasing aggression
   c) Enhancing alertness d) Promoting appetite

19. Cocaine affects animal behavior by primarily acting as a:
    a) Depressant b) Stimulant
    c) Sedative d) Hallucinogen
20. Which drug is known for its hallucinogenic effects on animal behavior?
    a) Alcohol b) Diazepam
    c) LSD (Lysergic acid diethylamide) d) Nicotine

Combined Hormones and Drugs Effects

21. Which hormone is released in response to stress and can influence the effects of drugs?
    a) Oxytocin b) Prolactin
    c) Cortisol d) Melatonin
22. Chronic use of which drug can alter dopamine levels and affect reward behavior?
    a) Nicotine b) Caffeine
    c) Cocaine d) Melatonin
23. What behavioral effect can high levels of cortisol have when combined with amphetamine use?
    a) Reduced aggression b) Increased stress and anxiety
    c) Enhanced sleep d) Decreased alertness
24. Which hormone can enhance the bonding effects of drugs like MDMA (Ecstasy)?
    a) Insulin b) Melatonin
    c) Oxytocin d) Prolactin
25. How can chronic alcohol consumption affect hormone levels related to stress?
    a) Increases oxytocin b) Decreases cortisol
    c) Increases cortisol d) Decreases melatonin
26. Which hormone, when elevated, can reduce the effects of stimulant drugs?
    a) Leptin b) Serotonin
    c) Ghrelin d) Prolactin
27. The interaction between nicotine and which hormone can influence appetite suppression?
    a) Estrogen b) Insulin
    c) Leptin d) Ghrelin
28. Increased levels of which neurotransmitter are often associated with the euphoric effects of drugs like cocaine and amphetamines?
    a) Serotonin b) Dopamine
    c) Melatonin d) Prolactin
29. Chronic stress and elevated cortisol levels can have what effect on the behavioral response to drugs?
    a) Enhance sedative effects b) Reduce anxiety
    c) Increase susceptibility to addiction d) Decrease aggressive behavior

30. The calming effects of benzodiazepines are primarily due to their interaction with which neurotransmitter?
    a) Dopamine
    b) GABA (Gamma-Aminobutyric Acid)
    c) Serotonin
    d) Norepinephrine

Hormones in Specific Animal Behaviors

31. Which hormone is critical for the seasonal migration behavior in birds?
    a) Testosterone b) Prolactin
    c) Melatonin d) Estrogen
32. In many mammals, which hormone facilitates the establishment of social hierarchies?
    a) Oxytocin b) Testosterone
    c) Cortisol d) Ghrelin
33. Which hormone is primarily involved in the regulation of parental care in male seahorses?
    a) Oxytocin b) Prolactin
    c) Cortisol d) Testosterone
34. Elevated levels of which hormone are associated with increased territorial behavior in fish?
    a) Estrogen b) Cortisol
    c) Testosterone d) Melatonin
35. In rodents, maternal behavior is significantly influenced by the release of which hormone?
    a) Oxytocin b) Ghrelin
    c) Insulin d) Adrenaline
36. Which hormone helps regulate hibernation behavior in bears?
    a) Leptin b) Melatonin
    c) Cortisol d) Ghrelin
37. In many bird species, courtship behavior is enhanced by which hormone?
    a) Oxytocin b) Prolactin
    c) Estrogen d) Melatonin
38. The fight-or-flight response is primarily mediated by which hormones?
    a) Serotonin and Melatonin b) Oxytocin and Prolactin
    c) Adrenaline and Noradrenaline d) Testosterone and Estrogen
39. Which hormone is responsible for regulating hunger and energy balance in animals?
    a) Insulin b) Leptin
    c) Oxytocin d) Prolactin

40. Which hormone is critical for the development of secondary sexual characteristics and mating behavior in male animals?
    a) Estrogen
    b) Progesterone
    c) Testosterone
    d) Cortisol

Drugs in Specific Animal Behaviors

41. Which drug is known to enhance exploratory behavior in animals?
    a) Alcohol
    b) Amphetamine
    c) Diazepam
    d) Morphine
42. What effect does morphine typically have on animal behavior?
    a) Increases alertness
    b) Induces pain relief and sedation
    c) Enhances aggression
    d) Stimulates appetite
43. Chronic use of which drug can lead to increased anxiety and stress behaviors in animals?
    a) Nicotine
    b) Caffeine
    c) Alcohol
    d) Cocaine
44. The calming effect of which drug makes it useful for treating anxiety in animals?
    a) Caffeine
    b) Diazepam (Valium)
    c) Nicotine
    d) Amphetamine
45. What effect does LSD typically have on animal behavior?
    a) Stimulant
    b) Depressant
    c) Hallucinogenic
    d) Sedative
46. Which drug is often used to study the effects of addiction and reward behavior in animals?
    a) Melatonin
    b) Cocaine
    c) Diazepam
    d) Morphine
47. The administration of which drug can help regulate sleep patterns in animals?
    a) Caffeine
    b) Melatonin
    c) Amphetamine
    d) Nicotine
48. How does chronic alcohol exposure affect animal behavior?
    a) Increases alertness
    b) Enhances memory
    c) Impairs coordination and increases aggression
    d) Reduces stress
49. Which drug can increase both locomotor activity and aggression in animals?
    a) Diazepam
    b) Cocaine
    c) Melatonin
    d) Alcohol

50. In research, which drug is often used to induce anxiety-like behaviors in animals?
    a) Caffeine
    b) Nicotine
    c) Corticosterone
    d) Diazepam

Interaction of Hormones and Drugs

51. High cortisol levels can interact with which drug to exacerbate anxiety?
    a) Diazepam
    b) Alcohol
    c) Amphetamine
    d) Melatonin
52. The combination of alcohol and high levels of which hormone can increase aggressive behavior?
    a) Oxytocin
    b) Melatonin
    c) Testosterone
    d) Leptin
53. Chronic stress can increase the susceptibility to addiction to which drug?
    a) Caffeine
    b) Nicotine
    c) Melatonin
    d) Diazepam
54. Elevated oxytocin levels can mitigate the anxiety effects of which drug?
    a) Cocaine
    b) Alcohol
    c) Amphetamine
    d) Diazepam
55. Which hormone can reduce the efficacy of stimulant drugs by promoting satiety?
    a) Ghrelin
    b) Leptin
    c) Insulin
    d) Estrogen
56. Chronic exposure to nicotine can alter the levels of which hormone associated with appetite regulation?
    a) Oxytocin
    b) Melatonin
    c) Ghrelin
    d) Leptin
57. The rewarding effects of drugs like amphetamines are primarily mediated by which neurotransmitter?
    a) Serotonin
    b) GABA
    c) Dopamine
    d) Acetylcholine
58. How does chronic stress affect the behavioral response to sedative drugs?
    a) Increases sedative effects
    b) Reduces susceptibility to addiction
    c) Enhances anxiety
    d) Reduces sedative effects
59. The interaction between benzodiazepines and which neurotransmitter results in calming effects?
    a) Dopamine
    b) Serotonin
    c) GABA
    d) Norepinephrine

60. Elevated serotonin levels can counteract the anxiety-inducing effects of which type of drug?
    a) Depressants b) Stimulants
    c) Hallucinogens d) Sedatives

Hormonal Effects in Various Species

61. In many fish species, increased testosterone levels during breeding season result in:
    a) Increased feeding behavior
    b) Decreased territoriality
    c) Increased aggression and territorial behavior
    d) Decreased mating behavior
62. Which hormone influences migratory restlessness in birds?
    a) Testosterone b) Prolactin
    c) Cortisol d) Melatonin
63. In primates, which hormone is crucial for maintaining social bonds and group cohesion?
    a) Insulin b) Oxytocin
    c) Adrenaline d) Ghrelin
64. Elevated levels of which hormone are associated with increased vocalization in male frogs during mating season?
    a) Melatonin b) Estrogen
    c) Testosterone d) Cortisol
65. In rodents, which hormone is linked to increased nesting behavior in preparation for offspring?
    a) Leptin b) Ghrelin
    c) Oxytocin d) Insulin
66. Which hormone helps regulate body fat and energy storage in animals preparing for hibernation?
    a) Cortisol b) Melatonin
    c) Leptin d) Ghrelin
67. In birds, the hormone prolactin is associated with which behavior?
    a) Migration b) Courtship
    c) Nest building and parental care d) Territorial aggression
68. What effect does elevated cortisol have on social hierarchies in primates?
    a) Reduces social bonding b) Increases cooperation
    c) Enhances maternal behavior d) Strengthens social bonds
69. Which hormone is crucial for the development of mating calls in male birds?
    a) Estrogen b) Prolactin
    c) Melatonin d) Testosterone

70. Increased levels of which hormone are linked to nurturing behaviors in male seahorses?
   a) Oxytocin
   b) Melatonin
   c) Prolactin
   d) Cortisol

Effects of Drugs in Various Species

71. Which drug is often used to reduce aggression in domestic animals?
   a) Caffeine
   b) Diazepam
   c) Amphetamine
   d) Nicotine
72. The use of which drug can increase stereotypic behaviors in animals, such as repetitive movements?
   a) Cocaine
   b) Alcohol
   c) Morphine
   d) Melatonin
73. What effect does chronic alcohol consumption have on social behavior in primates?
   a) Enhances social bonding
   b) Reduces social interactions
   c) Increases cooperation
   d) Decreases aggression
74. Which drug is commonly used to study the effects of depression in animal models?
   a) Diazepam
   b) Caffeine
   c) Corticosterone
   d) Amphetamine
75. How does chronic exposure to nicotine affect learning and memory in animals?
   a) Improves learning
   b) Has no effect
   c) Impairs memory
   d) Reduces stress
76. Which drug is known to cause hyperactivity and increased locomotion in rodents?
   a) Diazepam
   b) Melatonin
   c) Amphetamine
   d) Alcohol
77. The administration of which drug can induce sleep and reduce activity in animals?
   a) Nicotine
   b) Caffeine
   c) Melatonin
   d) Cocaine
78. Chronic stress can lead to increased self-administration of which drug in animal studies?
   a) Morphine
   b) Diazepam
   c) Alcohol
   d) Amphetamine
79. Which drug is often used to induce a state of analgesia and reduce pain in animals?
   a) Caffeine
   b) Nicotine
   c) Morphine
   d) Cocaine
80. What behavioral effect does LSD have on rodents in experimental settings?
   a) Reduces aggression
   b) Induces stereotypic behaviors
   c) Causes hallucinogenic-like behaviors
   d) Enhances memory

Answer Key

1	c	2	b	3	b	4	b	5	c	6	a	7	a
8	c	9	b	10	b	11	c	12	b	13	b	14	b
15	b	16	a	17	b	18	b	19	b	20	c	21	c
22	a	23	b	24	c	25	a	26	b	27	b	28	b
29	b	30	c										

Hormones and Animal Behavior

1	c	2	c	3	b	4	b	5	c	6	c	7	c
8	a	9	c	10	b	11	b	12	c	13	b	14	c
15	b	16	c	17	c	18	a	19	b	20	c		

Combined Hormones and Drugs Effects

21	c	22	c	23	b	24	c	25	c	26	b	27	c
28	b	29	c	30	b								

Hormones in Specific Animal Behaviors

31	c	32	b	33	b	34	c	35	a	36	b	37	c
38	c	39	b	40	c								

Drugs in Specific Animal Behaviors

41	b	42	b	43	d	44	b	45	c	46	b	47	b
48	c	49	b	50	c								

Interaction of Hormones and Drugs

51	c	52	c	53	b	54	a	55	b	56	d	57	c
58	d	59	c	60	b								

Hormonal Effects in Various Species

61	c	62	d	63	b	64	c	65	c	66	c	67	c
68	a	69	d	70	c								

Effects of Drugs in Various Species

71	b	72	a	73	b	74	c	75	c	76	c	77	c
78	d	79	c	80	c								

11

Ecology and Behavior

***Preeti Lakhani*[1], *Neeti Lakhani*[2] *and Ankita Rautella*[1]**

[1]*Department of Veterinary Physiology and Biochemistry, Lala Lajpat Rai University of Animal and Veterinary Sciences, Hsar, Harayana*

[2]*Department of Animal Nutrition, Guru Angad Deva University of Animal and Veterinary Sciences, Rampura Phool, Punjab*

Introduction

Ecological behavioral responses encompass a diverse array of adaptive behaviors exhibited by organisms in response to their dynamic environments. This interdisciplinary field integrates concepts from ecology and behavioral science to unravel the intricate ways in which organisms interact with and respond to their surroundings. This abstract provides a concise overview of key aspects within this burgeoning field.Firstly, behavioral responses to environmental stimuli are essential for the survival and reproduction of organisms. From foraging strategies and predator avoidance to mating rituals and territorial defense, the behaviors exhibited by individuals are often finely tuned to the ecological challenges they face. Understanding the mechanisms underlying these responses sheds light on the evolutionary processes shaping behavioral adaptations.Furthermore, the role of communication in ecological behavior cannot be overstated. Species communicate through a variety of means, including visual displays, vocalizations, chemical signals, and tactile interactions. These communication strategies facilitate intra and inter-species interactions, influencing mating choices, warning of potential threats, and establishing social hierarchies. Another critical aspect of ecological behavioral responses is the ability of organisms to adjust their behaviors in the face of environmental changes. Whether prompted by alterations in climate, resource availability, or human-induced disturbances, organisms exhibit plasticity in their behaviors. Such adaptability is crucial for species survival and underscores the importance of considering behavioral responses in conservation efforts and environmental management.Moreover, the study of behavioral responses provides valuable insights into ecosystem dynamics. Keystone species, which exert disproportionate influence on their ecosystems, often exhibit unique behavioral patterns that shape community structure and function. Investigating these behavioral interactions enhances our understanding of the intricate web of relationships that define ecological communities.In conclusion, ecological behavioral responses represent a multifaceted and dynamic area of study that deepens our understanding of how organisms navigate and thrive in their environments. By unraveling the complexities of behavior in an ecological context, researchers can contribute to more effective conservation strategies, improved ecosystem management, and a more holistic appreciation of the interconnectedness of life on Earth

MCQ's

1. What is the study of the relationships between organisms and their environments called?
   a) Geology b) Ecology
   c) Biology d) Meteorology
2. Which of the following is an abiotic factor in an ecosystem?
   a) Plants b) Animals
   c) Sunlight d) Bacteria
3. What is the primary source of energy in most ecosystems?
   a) Wind b) Sunlight
   c) Fossil fuels d) Geothermal heat
4. Which level of ecological organization includes all living organisms in a particular area?
   a) Population b) Community
   c) Ecosystem d) Biosphere
5. The process by which green plants use sunlight to synthesize food from carbon dioxide and water is known as:
   a) Respiration b) Photosynthesis
   c) Fermentation d) Digestion
6. What term is used to describe the maximum number of individuals of a species that an environment can support?
   a) Carrying capacity b) Biome capacity
   c) Population limit d) Habitat threshold
7. Which of the following is an example of a decomposer in an ecosystem?
   a) Rabbit b) Mushroom
   c) Eagle d) Snake
8. In the nitrogen cycle, bacteria play a crucial role in converting atmospheric nitrogen into a form that plants can use. This process is called:
   a) Nitrogen fixation b) Nitrogen assimilation
   c) Nitrification d) Denitrification
9. The loss of a species from a particular habitat is known as:
   a) Extinction b) Endangerment
   c) Extermination d) Exclusion
10. What is the term for the relationship where one organism benefits while the other is neither helped nor harmed?
    a) Mutualism b) Commensalism
    c) Parasitism d) Predation
11. Sexual selection is a type of natural selection that specifically acts on:
    a) Physical traits b) Behavioral traits
    c) Both physical and behavioral traits d) Environmental traits

12. Intrasexual selection involves competition:
    a) Between members of the same sex
    b) Between members of different species
    c) Between males and females
    d) Between predators and prey
13. The term "mate choice" refers to:
    a) Random pairing of individuals
    b) The process of finding a mate through fighting
    c) The selection of a mate based on certain traits
    d) Asexual reproduction
14. Which of the following is an example of an extravagant trait in males that may be favored by intersexual selection?
    a) Camouflage
    b) Bright plumage
    c) Aggressive behavior
    d) Speed
15. The concept of "sexy son hypothesis" suggests that females choose mates based on traits that will:
    a) Enhance their own survival
    b) Produce offspring with high genetic variability
    c) Increase the chances of their sons being attractive to females
    d) Ensure a high level of parental care from the male
16. Male-male competition for access to mates is often observed in species with:
    a) Monogamous mating systems
    b) Polyandrous mating systems
    c) Polygynous mating systems
    d) Asexual reproduction
17. What is the primary benefit of sexual selection?
    a) Increased genetic diversity
    b) Decreased competition
    c) Faster reproduction
    d) Greater energy efficiency
18. The peacock's elaborate tail feathers are an example of:
    a) Intrasexual selection
    b) Intersexual selection
    c) Natural selection
    d) A byproduct of evolution
19. The idea that female preferences for certain male traits can evolve based on indirect benefits, such as good genes, is known as:
    a) Handicap principle
    b) Direct benefits hypothesis
    c) Sexy son hypothesis
    d) Fisherian runaway selection
20. In many species, what is the role of courtship rituals in sexual selection?
    a) They serve no purpose in sexual selection
    b) They provide direct benefits to the female
    c) They help the female assess the genetic quality of the male
    d) They indicate the availability of mates to other males

21. Altruism in biology refers to behavior that:
    a) Benefits the individual exhibiting the behavior
    b) Benefits the recipient at a cost to the individual exhibiting the behavior
    c) Is harmful to both the individual and the recipient
    d) Has no impact on the fitness of the individuals involved
22. Kin selection is a theory that explains altruistic behavior by focusing on:
    a) Cooperation between unrelated individuals
    b) Cooperation within a social group
    c) Cooperation among individuals of different species
    d) Cooperation among close genetic relatives
23. Reciprocal altruism involves:
    a) Altruistic acts toward close kin
    b) Altruistic acts with the expectation of receiving a return favor
    c) Altruistic acts with no expectation of reciprocation
    d) Altruistic acts toward unrelated individuals
24. Inclusive fitness is a concept that combines:
    a) Personal fitness and environmental fitness
    b) Personal fitness and genetic fitness
    c) Genetic fitness and environmental fitness
    d) Personal fitness, genetic fitness, and reproductive fitness
25. Eusociality is a form of social organization characterized by:
    a) Competition among group members
    b) Altruistic behavior, reproductive division of labor, and cooperative care of offspring
    c) Territorial aggression
    d) Isolation and independence among individuals
26. Which of the following is an example of altruism in the animal kingdom?
    a) A lion hunting for its prey
    b) Bees sacrificing themselves to defend the hive
    c) A cheetah chasing down its prey
    d) A wolf marking its territory
27. According to the "reciprocal altruism" hypothesis, altruistic behavior is likely to evolve in:
    a) Isolated populations with little interaction
    b) Large populations with intense competition
    c) Small, closely-knit groups where individuals interact repeatedly
    d) Species with low reproductive rates

28. The concept of "altruistic punishment" suggests that individuals may punish others for:
    a) Their own benefit
    b) The benefit of the group
    c) Altruistic acts
    d) Selfish behavior
29. Altruism can be challenging to explain from an evolutionary perspective because:
    a) Altruistic behaviors are always maladaptive
    b) Altruistic behaviors rarely occur in nature
    c) Altruistic behaviors often reduce an individual's reproductive success
    d) Altruistic behaviors only occur in highly intelligent species
30. "Tit for tat" is a strategy associated with:
    a) Kin selection
    b) Reciprocal altruism
    c) Eusociality
    d) Altruistic punishment
31. Which of the following is an example of a benefit derived from social behavior in animals?
    a) Increased competition for resources
    b) Enhanced survival and reproductive success
    c) Isolation from the group
    d) Decreased communication within the group
32. The term "allogrooming" refers to:
    a) Aggressive behavior within a social group
    b) Mutual grooming between individuals
    c) Solitary grooming behavior
    d) Territorial marking
33. In a dominance hierarchy, individuals establish and maintain their social status through:
    a) Random interactions
    b) Aggressive displays
    c) Cooperative hunting
    d) Altruistic behavior
34. Cooperative breeding is a social behavior where:
    a) Offspring are raised by a single parent
    b) Offspring are cared for by individuals other than the biological parents
    c) There is no parental care for the offspring
    d) Mating occurs within family groups
35. The term "territoriality" in social behavior refers to:
    a) Migration patterns within a species
    b) The defense of a specific area against others of the same species
    c) The avoidance of social interactions
    d) The random distribution of individuals within a habitat
36. Communication is a crucial aspect of social behavior in animals. Which of the following is a common form of animal communication?
    a) Verbal language
    b) Written messages
    c) Chemical signals
    d) Morse code

37. What is the primary advantage of living in social groups for animals?
    a) Increased competition for resources
    b) Enhanced defense against predators
    c) Reduced reproductive success
    d) Isolation from disease
38. The "selfish herd" concept suggests that individuals in a group benefit from:
    a) Increased competition within the group
    b) Forming larger groups for protection against predators
    c) Isolation from other groups
    d) Decreased communication within the group
39. What is the term for the phenomenon where individuals in a group take turns being at the front, reducing the energy required for long-distance travel?
    a) Leadership rotation b) Social cycling
    c) Pack migration d) Drafting
40. What is communication in animals primarily used for?
    a) Obtaining food b) Attracting mates
    c) Establishing dominance d) All of the above
41. Chemical signals, such as pheromones, are commonly used for:
    a) Long-distance communication b) Visual displays
    c) Auditory communication d) Tactile communication
42. In the context of animal communication, what does the term "cue" refer to?
    a) A specific signal that elicits a response b) A type of vocalization
    c) A physical gesture d) A visual display
43. The waggle dance in honeybees is a form of communication used for:
    a) Attracting mates b) Warning of danger
    c) Navigating to a food source d) Establishing dominance
44. Which sense is often involved in visual communication in animals?
    a) Smell b) Hearing
    c) Sight d) Taste
45. What is the primary function of territorial signals in animals?
    a) Attracting mates b) Warning intruders
    c) Establishing dominance d) Navigating to a food source
46. The term "agonistic behavior" is associated with communication related to:
    a) Reproduction b) Aggression and conflict
    c) Territory marking d) Food acquisition
47. Vocalizations in animals are commonly used for:
    a) Attracting mates b) Establishing territory
    c) Warning of danger d) All of the above

48. Echolocation is a form of communication primarily used by:
    a) Birds b) Bats
    c) Insects d) Fish
49. What is mimicry in the context of animal communication?
    a) Imitating the signals of other species
    b) Producing random signals
    c) Non-voluntary communication
    d) Ignoring communication signals
50. What is the term for the study of the physiological mechanisms underlying animal behavior?
    a) Ethology b) Psychology
    c) Behaviorology d) Behavioral physiology
51. The endocrine system is responsible for the release of:
    a) Electrical signals b) Hormones
    c) Neurotransmitters d) Enzymes
52. In the context of behavior physiology, what role do neurotransmitters play?
    a) Regulating hormone production
    b) Transmitting signals between nerve cells
    c) Controlling muscular movements
    d) Enhancing sensory perception
53. The hypothalamus is a key brain region involved in:
    a) Memory formation b) Emotional processing
    c) Hormone regulation d) Muscle coordination
54. Which of the following hormones is often associated with the "fight or flight" response?
    a) Insulin b) Adrenaline (epinephrine)
    c) Estrogen d) Testosterone
55. How do sensory receptors contribute to behavior physiology?
    a) By producing hormones
    b) By transmitting signals to the brain
    c) By regulating muscle contractions
    d) By controlling body temperature
56. The process by which an animal's behavior is influenced by past experiences and learned associations is known as:
    a) Innate behavior b) Classical conditioning
    c) Operant conditioning d) Instinctive behavior
57. In Pavlov's classical conditioning experiments, what did the dog initially learn to associate with food?
    a) A bell b) A light
    c) A sound d) A specific location

58. How does the circadian rhythm influence behavior in animals?
  a) It regulates hormone production
  b) It affects sleep-wake cycles and activity levels
  c) It controls muscle coordination
  d) It influences reproductive behavior

59. Which brain structure is often associated with the regulation of emotions and emotional responses?
  a) Cerebellum b) Amygdala
  c) Medulla oblongata d) Hippocampus

60. What is the term for the zone of the ocean where sunlight can penetrate and photosynthesis can occur?
  a) Hadal zone b) Abyssal zone
  c) Epipelagic zone d) Bathypelagic zone

61. Which factor is a key determinant of water quality in aquatic ecosystems?
  a) Water temperature b) Air pressure
  c) Soil composition d) Wind speed

62. The term "eutrophication" refers to:
  a) The depletion of nutrients in aquatic ecosystems
  b) The excessive growth of algae and plants due to nutrient enrichment
  c) The migration of fish species
  d) The formation of coral reefs

63. What is a primary source of oxygen production in aquatic ecosystems?
  a) Algae and phytoplankton b) Fish & other aquatic animals
  c) Sedimentation d) Bacteria

64. Which type of wetland is characterized by waterlogged soils and is often dominated by cattails and sedges?
  a) Marsh b) Swamp
  c) Bog d) Fen

65. The process of desalination is most commonly used to:
  a) Increase salt concentration in seawater
  b) Reduce salt concentration in seawater
  c) Eliminate algae in freshwater ecosystems
  d) Promote the growth of aquatic plants

66. What is the main factor contributing to coral bleaching in coral reefs?
  a) Pollution b) Overfishing
  c) Ocean acidification d) Elevated water temperatures

67. The oxygen minimum zone (OMZ) is characterized by:
  a) High concentrations of dissolved oxygen
  b) Low concentrations of dissolved oxygen
  c) High levels of salinity
  d) Low levels of salinity

68. An estuary is a unique aquatic habitat where:
    a) Freshwater and saltwater mix
    b) Only freshwater is present
    c) Only saltwater is present
    d) There is no plant life

69. Which of the following is a common pollutant that can have detrimental effects on aquatic ecosystems?
    a) Oxygen
    b) Nitrogen
    c) Phosphorus
    d) Carbon dioxide

70. What is cooperation in ecology?
    a) Competition between individuals of the same species
    b) Interaction between individuals that benefits both
    c) Aggressive behavior within a population
    d) A form of symbiosis

71. Mutualism is an example of cooperation where:
    a) One organism benefits, and the other is harmed
    b) Both organisms benefit
    c) One organism benefits at the expense of the other
    d) There is no interaction between organisms

72. The sharing of resources within a group to reduce the risk of predation is an example of:
    a) Competition
    b) Altruism
    c) Cooperative hunting
    d) Mutualism

73. Eusociality, as observed in colonies of ants and bees, involves:
    a) Solitary behavior
    b) Cooperative care of offspring and reproductive division of labor
    c) Aggressive behavior
    d) Competitive interactions

74. In a classic example of cooperation, oxpecker birds feed on parasites found on the bodies of large mammals, such as buffaloes. This is an example of:
    a) Commensalism
    b) Mutualism
    c) Parasitism
    d) Predation

75. How does kin selection contribute to cooperative behavior in animals?
    a) By favoring the survival and reproduction of close relatives
    b) By promoting competition within families
    c) By reducing cooperation between unrelated individuals
    d) By minimizing the role of genetics in behavior

76. The behavior where individuals warn others of potential danger, even at a personal cost, is known as:
    a) Aggression
    b) Altruism
    c) Competition
    d) Predation

77. What is the term for a cooperative behavior where individuals take turns in a specific role or position?
   a) Dominance hierarchy
   b) Reciprocal altruism
   c) Tit-for-tat strategy
   d) Task specialization

78. Cleaner fish, such as the cleaner wrasse, engage in mutualistic interactions by:
   a) Feeding on parasites on larger fish
   b) Preying on larger fish
   c) Competing for resources with larger fish
   d) Avoiding interactions with larger fish

79. Cooperative breeding involves:
   a) A single parent raising offspring
   b) Offspring being cared for by individuals other than the parents
   c) No parental care for the offspring
   d) Mating within family groups

80. What does "behavioral plasticity" refer to in the context of animal behavior?
   a) Rigidity and inflexibility in behavior
   b) The ability of an organism to change its behavior in response to environmental cues
   c) Fixed and genetically determined behaviors
   d) The absence of behavioral responses

81. Which of the following is an example of behavioral plasticity?
   a) A genetically determined courtship display in birds
   b) A fish changing its foraging behavior in response to food availability
   c) A spider building a web using a genetically preset pattern
   d) A bird singing the same song throughout its life

82. Phenotypic plasticity refers to the ability of an organism to:
   a) Produce offspring with different phenotypes
   b) Adjust its phenotype in response to environmental conditions
   c) Exhibit fixed and unchanging traits
   d) Avoid environmental changes

83. The ability of an animal to learn from experience and modify its behavior accordingly is known as:
   a) Fixed action pattern
   b) Habituation
   c) Classical conditioning
   d) Behavioral rigidity

84. Which of the following is an example of habituation?
   a) A dog learning to associate a bell with food
   b) A bird changing its feeding behavior after encountering a new food source
   c) A cat exhibiting a fixed hunting pattern
   d) A fish displaying a courtship behavior when introduced to a new mate

85. In the context of behavioral ecology, how does "phenotypic plasticity" contribute to an organism's fitness?
   a) It ensures that the organism always exhibits the same behavior.
   b) It allows the organism to adjust its behavior to maximize survival and reproduction in different environments.
   c) It limits the adaptability of the organism to changing conditions.
   d) It results in the loss of genetic diversity.

86. A behavior that is genetically determined and expressed in response to a specific stimulus is known as a:
   a) Flexible behavior b) Fixed action pattern
   c) Phenotypic plasticity d) Non-responsive behavior

87. Which of the following factors can influence behavioral plasticity?
   a) Genetic makeup b) Environmental conditions
   c) Learning experiences d) All of the above

88. An animal that adjusts its activity pattern based on daily fluctuations in temperature is exhibiting:
   a) Classical conditioning b) Behavioral rigidity
   c) Circadian rhythms d) Phenotypic plasticity

89. "Neuroplasticity" refers to the brain's ability to:
   a) Maintain a fixed structure throughout an organism's life
   b) Change and reorganize in response to experience
   c) Exhibit rigid and inflexible behavior
   d) Resist any changes in neural connections

90. Natural selection is based on:
   a) Human intervention b) Random chance
   c) Differential reproductive success d) Genetic mutations

91. Which of the following is a requirement for natural selection to occur?
   a) Large population size b) Genetic variation
   c) Lack of environmental changes d) Short generation time

92. In the context of evolution, what does "fitness" refer to?
   a) Physical strength b) Ability to survive and reproduce
   c) Adaptability to the environment d) Number of offspring produced

93. What type of selection favors extreme phenotypes in a population?
   a) Stabilizing selection b) Disruptive selection
   c) Directional selection d) Artificial selection

94. In sexual selection, traits that enhance an individual's attractiveness to the opposite sex are known as:
   a) Adaptive traits b) Dominant traits
   c) Secondary sexual characteristics d) Neutral traits

95. Which scientist is credited with proposing the theory of natural selection independently of Charles Darwin?

a) Gregor Mendel
b) Alfred Russel Wallace
c) Thomas Malthus
d) Jean-Baptiste Lamarck

96. Artificial selection is a process where:

a) Natural forces drive evolution
b) Humans selectively breed organisms for desirable traits
c) Random mutations determine trait variation
d) Evolution occurs without any selection pressures

97. In directional selection, what happens to the frequency of a particular trait over time?

a) It decreases
b) It remains constant
c) It increases
d) It fluctuates randomly

98. What is the main difference between natural selection and artificial selection?

a) Natural selection is driven by humans, while artificial selection occurs in the wild
b) Artificial selection is slower than natural selection
c) Natural selection is a natural process, while artificial selection is driven by human intervention
d) Both processes are identical

99. Selective pressures that lead to the evolution of similar traits in unrelated species are known as:

a) Convergent evolution
b) Divergent evolution
c) Coevolution
d) Parallel evolution

100. In a prey-predator relationship, the organism that hunts and kills another organism for food is the:

a) Prey
b) Predator
c) Consumer
d) Producer

101. Mimicry in prey species is an adaptation that serves to:

a) Attract predators
b) Confuse predators
c) Increase predation risk
d) Camouflage the prey

102. What is the term for the phenomenon where a harmless species evolves to resemble a harmful or poisonous species to avoid predation?

a) Camouflage
b) Batesian mimicry
c) Mutualism
d) Warning coloration

103. The concept of coevolution in prey-predator relationships suggests that:

a) Predators always evolve faster than prey
b) Prey and predators evolve independently of each other
c) Evolutionary changes in one species lead to reciprocal changes in the other
d) Predators are not influenced by the traits of their prey

104. Aposematism refers to:
   a) Mimicry in prey
   b) Warning coloration in prey
   c) Camouflage in predators
   d) Aggressive behavior in predators

105. Which type of prey-predator relationship benefits both the predator and prey involved?
   a) Parasitism
   b) Mutualism
   c) Competition
   d) Commensalism

106. What is the primary reason for the evolution of cryptic coloration in prey species?
   a) To warn predators
   b) To attract mates
   c) To hide from predators
   d) To signal aggression

107. A population of rabbits increasing in size due to abundant food and low predation is an example of:
   a) Commensalism
   b) Symbiosis
   c) Predator-prey cycle
   d) Competitive exclusion

108. The Lotka-Volterra equations are used to model:
   a) Mutualistic relationships
   b) Predator-prey interactions
   c) Commensalism
   d) Competition between species

109. A secondary compound produced by a plant that makes it unpalatable or toxic to herbivores is an example of:
   a) Batesian mimicry
   b) Aposematism
   c) Chemical defense
   d) Mutualism

110. What is Batesian mimicry?
   a) Both species involved benefit from the mimicry
   b) The mimic is harmful, and the model is harmless
   c) The mimic and model are both harmful
   d) The mimic resembles an inanimate object

111. Müllerian mimicry involves:
   a) Harmful species resembling each other
   b) A harmless species resembling a harmful species
   c) A predator mimicking its prey
   d) The mimicry of sounds and vocalizations

112. Which type of mimicry involves an organism resembling its surroundings to avoid detection by predators or prey?
   a) Müllerian mimicry
   b) Batesian mimicry
   c) Cryptic mimicry
   d) Aggressive mimicry

113. In aggressive mimicry, an organism mimics:
   a) A harmful model to avoid predation
   b) Its prey to facilitate predation
   c) An inanimate object for protection
   d) The appearance of a mate for reproductive success

114. What is automimicry or intraspecific mimicry?
  a) Mimicry between different species
  b) Mimicry within the same species
  c) Mimicry involving multiple species
  d) Mimicry involving only females

115. A harmless viceroy butterfly mimicking the appearance of a toxic monarch butterfly is an example of:
  a) Müllerian mimicry
  b) Batesian mimicry
  c) Cryptic mimicry
  d) Automimicry

116. Aggressive mimicry is most commonly observed in:
  a) Predatory animals
  b) Herbivorous animals
  c) Prey animals
  d) Animals with warning coloration

117. What is protective mimicry?
  a) Mimicry to deceive predators
  b) Mimicry for reproductive success
  c) Mimicry to gain protection from a mutualistic partner
  d) Mimicry to attract mates

118. Which type of mimicry involves an organism mimicking a harmful or toxic model to gain protection?
  a) Cryptic mimicry
  b) Batesian mimicry
  c) Automimicry
  d) Müllerian mimicry

119. In crypsis, an organism mimics:
  a) A harmful model
  b) Its prey
  c) Its surroundings
  d) Other members of its species

120. What does cognition refer to?
  a) Physical abilities
  b) Mental processes and activities related to knowledge
  c) Communication skills
  d) Behavioral responses to stimuli

121. In the context of animal cognition, what is meant by "theory of mind"?
  a) The ability to understand one's own thoughts and emotions
  b) The ability to understand the thoughts and emotions of others
  c) The process of forming theories about the environment
  d) The ability to navigate and create mental maps

122. Communication involves the exchange of information between individuals. What is a key component of communication in animals?
  a) Telepathy
  b) Body language
  c) Abstract symbols
  d) Inaudible sounds

123. In animal communication, what is a pheromone?
  a) A visual signal
  b) A chemical signal
  c) An auditory signal
  d) A tactile signal

124. Which of the following is an example of non-verbal communication in humans?
 a) Speaking b) Writing
 c) Facial expressions d) Sign language
125. What is the primary purpose of alarm calls in the animal kingdom?
 a) Attracting mates b) Signaling aggression
 c) Warning others about potential danger d) Establishing territory
126. Which of the following is an example of a complex cognitive ability in animals?
 a) Associative learning b) Reflex actions
 c) Fixed action patterns d) Instinctive behaviors
127. What is the role of mimicry in communication?
 a) To confuse predators b) To attract mates
 c) To establish dominance d) To signal submission
128. In animal communication, what is "ritualization"?
 a) The use of rituals for communication
 b) The process of refining and simplifying signals for communication
 c) The use of body language exclusively
 d) The development of complex vocalizations
129. Which of the following is an example of a symbolic communication system in animals?
 a) Bee dances b) Bird songs
 c) Dolphin clicks d) Human language
130. What is the role of the hypothalamus in neuroendocrine regulation?
 a) Regulation of body temperature
 b) Production of hormones
 c) Coordination of voluntary movements
 d) Integration of nervous and endocrine systems
131. Which gland is often referred to as the "master gland" because it controls the functions of other endocrine glands?
 a) Thyroid gland b) Adrenal gland
 c) Pituitary gland d) Pancreas
132. The release of adrenaline during the "fight or flight" response is an example of neuroendocrine regulation by the:
 a) Pituitary gland b) Thyroid gland
 c) Adrenal gland d) Pancreas
133. What is the primary function of the thyroid gland in neuroendocrine regulation?
 a) Regulation of blood sugar levels
 b) Regulation of metabolism and energy production
 c) Regulation of calcium levels in the blood
 d) Regulation of the sleep-wake cycle

134. The pineal gland is responsible for the production of which hormone that regulates the sleep-wake cycle?
   a) Melatonin
   b) Insulin
   c) Cortisol
   d) Epinephrine
135. How does the endocrine system contribute to the regulation of reproductive behavior in animals?
   a) By controlling muscle coordination
   b) By regulating water balance
   c) By influencing the release of sex hormones
   d) By mediating the sense of smell
136. The release of oxytocin during childbirth and lactation is an example of neuroendocrine regulation in:
   a) Matingbehavior
   b) Parental care
   c) Social bonding
   d) Thermoregulation
137. In seasonal breeders, such as many mammals, the reproductive cycle is often influenced by changes in:
   a) Light and temperature
   b) Food availability
   c) Water balance
   d) Social interactions
138. What is the role of corticosteroids in the stress response within the neuroendocrine system?
   a) Stimulating growth hormone production
   b) Promoting immune system function
   c) Reducing inflammation
   d) Regulating blood pressure
139. How do pheromones contribute to neuroendocrine regulation in animal behavior?
   a) By influencing the release of sex hormones
   b) By regulating body temperature
   c) By promoting sleep
   d) By controlling water balance
140. What is the main focus of genetic ecology?
   a) Studying the behavior of organisms
   b) Investigating the impact of climate change on ecosystems
   c) Understanding the genetic basis of ecological processes
   d) Analyzing the physical structure of ecosystems
141. How does genetic diversity contribute to the adaptability of a population to environmental changes?
   a) By reducing the chances of mutation
   b) By limiting the range of available traits
   c) By increasing the likelihood of survival and reproduction
   d) By decreasing the rate of genetic recombination

142. Which term refers to the variety of alleles present in a population at a particular genetic locus?

a) Genotype
b) Phenotype
c) Heterozygosity
d) Allelic diversity

143. The Hardy-Weinberg equilibrium is a principle used in genetic ecology to:

a) Predict changes in allele frequencies over generations
b) Assess the impact of climate change on ecosystems
c) Measure the size of a population
d) Identify invasive species

144. What is gene flow in the context of genetic ecology?

a) The movement of genes between populations
b) The exchange of genetic material between generations
c) The elimination of specific genes from a population
d) The process of genetic mutation

145. A population bottleneck can lead to:

a) Increased genetic diversity
b) Decreased genetic diversity
c) Stable genetic composition
d) Enhanced adaptability

146. Which factor contributes to the founder effect in genetic ecology?

a) Large population size
b) Random mating patterns
c) Migration of individuals
d) Establishment of a new population by a small group

147. Genetic drift is most influential in:

a) Largepopulations
b) Small populations
c) Populations with high gene flow
d) Populations with low mutation rates

148. How does natural selection influence the genetic makeup of a population?

a) By promoting the survival of individuals with certain traits
b) By preventing genetic mutations
c) By eliminating genetic diversity
d) By increasing the rate of genetic drift

149. Which term describes the occurrence of two or more alleles at a particular locus in a population?

a) Monogenic
b) Polygenic
c) Polymorphism
d) Homozygosity

150. In classical conditioning, what is paired to create a learned association?
  a) A stimulus and a response
  b) Two neutral stimuli
  c) A conditioned stimulus and an unconditioned stimulus
  d) Two conditioned responses

Answer Key

1	b	2	c	3	b	4	c	5	b	6	a	7	b
8	a	9	a	10	b	11	c	12	a	13	c	14	b
15	c	16	c	17	a	18	b	19	d	20	c	21	b
22	d	23	b	24	b	25	b	26	b	27	c	28	b
29	c	30	b	31	b	32	b	33	b	34	b	35	b
36	c	37	b	38	b	39	d	40	d	41	a	42	a
43	c	44	c	45	b	46	b	47	d	48	b	49	a
50	d	51	b	52	b	53	c	54	b	55	b	56	c
57	a	58	b	59	b	60	c	61	a	62	b	63	a
64	a	65	b	66	d	67	b	68	a	69	c	70	b
71	b	72	c	73	b	74	a	75	a	76	b	77	c
78	a	79	b	80	b	81	b	82	b	83	b	84	b
85	b	86	b	87	d	88	c	89	b	90	c	91	b
92	b	93	c	94	c	95	b	96	b	97	c	98	c
99	c	100	b	101	b	102	b	103	c	104	b	105	b
106	c	107	c	108	b	109	c	110	b	111	a	112	c
113	b	114	b	115	b	116	a	117	a	118	b	119	c
120	b	121	b	122	b	123	b	124	c	125	c	126	a
127	a	128	b	129	d	130	d	131	c	132	c	133	b
134	a	135	c	136	c	137	a	138	c	139	a	140	c
141	c	142	c	143	a	144	a	145	b	146	d	147	b
148	a	149	c	150	c								

12

Social Dominance and Territoriality

Cherryl D. Miranda[1] and Vallabhaneni Srikanth[2]

[1]*Department of Livestock Production Management, Veterinary College, Athani Karnataka Veterinary, Animal and Fisheries Sciences University, Bidar, Karnataka*

[2]*Livestock Production & Management Section, ICAR-Indian Veterinary Research Institute (ICAR-IVRI), Izatnagar, Bareilly, Uttar Pradesh*

Introduction

An animal's asymmetry in aggression towards another species is commonly used to characterise its dominance. In other contexts, dominance describes people who emerge victorious from brief dyadic competitions. Most animal groups are arranged in a hierarchical fashion, whereby members at higher ranks have more access to resources and opportunity for procreation than members at lower ranks.

Signals of Dominance: Acts or structures known as signals are employed by signalers to convey information to recipients in a way that elicits a response from them. This response usually has positive fitness consequences for both the signaler and the recipient. These signs don't always have to be easy to see.

Communities vary in the hierarchical pattern of dominance. The most common kind of rank relationships are those in which there is a "alpha" who is better than all other members of the group, a "beta" who is better than all members except the "alpha," and so on down the hierarchy to the lowest ranker who is under all others. Therefore, if powerful males may be arranged in a single sequence, the system is known as a simple and linear dominance hierarchy.

Concepts of Dominance Hierarchies

1. Establishing dominance
2. Maintaining dominance

Dominance Hierarchy Types

1. Statistical hierarchy
2. Confidence hierarchy
3. Assessment hierarchy

For those who live in tiny groups, maintaining stable dominance is extremely crucial. Social instability has a negative effect on animal survivorship, reproductive success, longevity, stress reactivity, weaning percentage, and weight gain in young animals. Individual animals in the lower ranks of unstable societies will sometimes test their dominating peers by acting aggressively, believing that this will help them advance in their status.

Territoriality

Animals exhibit a complex phenomenon called territoriality that is engrained in their behavioural repertoire.

Evolutionary Significance of Territoriality

- Resource Partitioning
- Reproductive Success
- Population Regulation

Mechanisms of Territorial Defense

1. Physical Defense
2. Vocalizations and Displays
3. Chemical Signaling
4. Territorial Boundaries

Exclusive Territories: These areas are guarded by one individual or a group of individuals against any invaders.

Overlap Territories: Overlap territories are areas where the territories of multiple individuals or groups intersect.

Usually males mark their territories before breeding, and during breeding season, defence is heightened, especially between males of the same species.

Classification of territories: Territories in relation to birds have been classified by Nice (1941) into several basic types:

a) Entire mating, feeding, and breeding area defended. Eg. Song Sparrow
b) Mating and nesting but not feeding area defended. Eg. Scarlet Finch
c) Mating area only defended. Eg. Gould's Manakin
d) Nest only defended. Eg. Night Heron
e) Winter territories. Eg. Black-bellied Plover
f) Roosting territories. Eg. Starling, Tree Creepe

Territorial behaviour serves multiple functions crucial for an animal's survival and reproductive success like resource acquisition, mate attraction, defense, protection of offspring, status and social structure.

1. Social structure in a group is completely dependent on
   a) Dominance hierarchy
   b) Dominance ordinate hierarcy
   c) Dominance subordinate hierarcy
   d) Ordinate hierarcy
2. Which among the following may have impact on hierarcy development
   a) Social norms
   b) Social dynamics
   c) Both
   d) None
3. When does this social dominance relationship exists among most of the individuals
   a) Limited resources
   b) Incompatability
   c) Plenty resources
   d) Both a and b

4. Excel in short-term dyadic competitions describes
   a) Dominance   b) Co-dominance
   c) Dependency   d Inter
5. Predominate factor that influences the social dominance
   a) Weight   b) Age
   c) Both a and b   d) Size
6. Age is considered as positively correlated with social dominace in
   a) Sheep   b) Goat
   c) Both a and b   d) Horse
7. Weight is considered as positively correlated to social dominace in
   a) Sheep   b) Horse
   c) Goat   d) Buffalo
8. Among the following which is the fundamental aspect of animal behaviour
   a) Territoriality   b) Terrestriality
   c) Both   d) None
9. Asymmetry in aggression by one animal towards another animal is defined as
   a) Dependency   b) Co-dominance
   c) dominance   d) Inter-dependency
10. Following are the random structures that communicates status signals and are inexpensive to make
   a) Signal status   b) Badges of status
   c) Signalling   d) None
11. Numerous social groupings feature hierarchies of dominance that are
   a) Linear   b) Non linear
   c) Curvilinear   d) Bell shaped
12. The hierarcical structures of dominace differs among
   a) Groups   b) Classes
   c) Communities   d) All
13. Superior to every member of the group
   a) Beta   b) Alpha
   c) Gamma   d) Delta
14. Concept that is Imporatant in dominance hierarchies
   a) Establishing dominance   b) Maintaining dominance
   c) Both   d) None
15. Fundamental forms of dominance hierarchies have been identified by
   a) Barnard and Burk   b) Tibbetts
   c) Burk   d) Drews

16. Which type of dominance hierarchy is uncommon in nature
    a) Statistica b) Confidence
    c) Assessment d) Temporal
17. Mechanisms that keep hierarchies stable are
    a) Variety of behaviours b) Society set up
    c) None d) Both a and b
18. Behaviours used by dominants to punish their subordinates are
    a) Aggression b) Infanticide
    c) Eviction d) All
19. Individual recognition is the most popular method for determining
    a) Sub-ordinate position b) Dominance position
    c) Both d) None
20. In many stable bird flocks individual recognition is through
    a) Call b) Plumage
    c) None d) Both
21. For individually identify group members, primates use information from their
    a) Smell b) Sound
    c) Sight d) All
22. Kinship and rank are used incase of
    a) Baboons b) Monkey
    c) Birds d) Reptiles
23. Trustworthy signals of dominance exhibit
    a) Phenotypic changes b) Genotypic changes
    c) Both d) None
24. A simple method that requires little cognitive work to quickly and accurately determine dominance rank is
    a) Interactions b) Signals
    c) Both d) None
25. In swine individual dominance relationships are established before
    a) 9 weeks b) 10weeks
    c) 8 weeks d) 7 weeks
26. In calves the ranking order is established between
    a) 3-6 months b) 2-4 months
    c) 4-6 months d) 4-8 months
27. Social dominance indicates
    a) Rank b) Degree of differences
    c) Both d) None
28. Dominance development is a
    a) Innate b) Learned
    c) Both d) None

29. Control mechanism for the social organisation
    a) Nteractions b) Co-dominance
    c) Inter-dominance d) Dominance
30. Area held and defended by group of organisms is called
    a) Territory b) Territoriality
    c) Both d) None
31. Groups keep members of the same species from invading a space region - given by
    a) Ardrey b) Brower
    c) Altman d) Taylor
32. It is an action taken either temporarily or permanently to stop others from using the areas and items- given by
    a) Brown b) Brower
    c) Taylor d) Altman
33. A persons outward manifestation of their sense of possession over a material or social object
    a) Ardrey b) Brown
    c) Taylor d) Altman
34. Vertebrates as well as higher invertebrates confine their activities to a certain region known as
    a) Home tract b) Home zone
    c) Home region d) Home range
35. Territories can be categorized into........ groups
    a) 2 b) 3
    c) 4 d) 5
36. Territories defended against all intruders,typicall by a single individual or a group
    a) Overlap territories b) Inclusive territories
    c) Exclusive territories d) Mutual territories
37. Areas where the territories of multiple individuals or groups intersect
    a) Overlap territories b) Inclusive territories
    c) Exclusive territories d) Mutual territories
38. The dimensions of territory and the extent of the home range typically diminsh as population density
    a) Decreases b) Increases
    c) Does not changes d) Both a and b
39. In vertebrates territoriality is particularly noticeable because
    a) Sexual behaviour b) Ingestive behaviour
    c) Agonistic behaviour d) Reproductive behaviour

40. Most of the time territorial behaviour is limited to the..........season
   a) Mating b) Summer
   c) Spring d) Monsoon
41. Territory formation .... habit utilization
   a) Maximizing b) Minimizing
   c) Does not affects d) Both a and b
42. Territories are established predominantly by
   a) Females b) Males
   c) Any one of the sex d) Both the sex
43. Territory acquisition primarily involves .... rather than physical combat
   a) Threats b) Gestures
   c) Postures d) All
44. Territories in relation to birds have been classified by
   a) Altman b) Taylor
   c) Nice d) Brown
45. Primary functions of territoriality
   a) Mate attraction and defense b) Resource acquistion
   c) Protection of offspring d) All
46. Individuals use territories to display their quality or fitness to potential mates through
   a) Courtship display b) Territorial defense
   c) Both d) None
47. Mechanism of territorial defense includes
   a) Physical defense b) Vocalization
   c) Chemical signaling d) All
48. Visual displays to advertise ownership and intimidate rivals
   a) Posturing b) Territorial markings
   c) Both d) None
49. Which of the following will reduces the likelihood of territorial disputes
   a) Chemical signaling b) Territorial boundaries
   c) Vocalizations d) Physical defense
50. Resource partitioning promotes
   a) Species coexistence b) Niche differentiation
   c) Reducing competition d) All
51. Canine territoraial markings encompass
   a) Olfactory b) Visual
   c) Both d) Vocalization

52. In regions with winter snowfall urination sites are recognizable as
    a) Yellow snow b) Dark snow
    c) Pale snow d) Scent snow
53. Cattle display territorial aggression through acts such as
    a) Running b) Butting
    c) Bellowing d) Bleating
54. Horses exhibits territorial aggression by utilizing
    a) Offensive tactics b) Defensive tactics
    c) Both d) None
55. In the grazing territories of horse the cropped areas known as
    a) Roughs b) Greens
    c) Feeds d) Lawns
56 In the grazing territories of horse the dung areas known as
    a) Roughs b) Heeps
    c) Dirt d) Dung land
57. In the grazing territories of horse areas left untouched except during scarcity of food resources
    a) Lawns b) Heeps
    c) Roughs d) Roughages
58. Incase of sheep in the absence of a submissive reaction, they might
    a) Tug b) Push
    c) Butt at wool d) All
59. Intensive contact behaviour is seen mostly in
    a) Cattle b) Sheep
    c) Goat d) Pig
60. Very little territorialism is mostly seen in
    a) Cattl b) Pig
    c) Goat d) Sheep
61. Among the following strategies to defend their territory which is proved to be suboptimal
    a) Vocalization b) Visual display
    c) Fighting d) Odors
62. Which method effectively deters approaching animals without the need for direct conforntation with the territory's defender
    a) Use scent markings b) Vocalization
    c) Visual display d) Physical defense
63. Territorial marking system occasionally seen in females of
    a) Dogs b) Cats
    c) Pig d) Horse

64. Territories will have____________ boundaries
   a) Circular b) Hexagonal
   c) Pentagonal d) Octagonal
65. Economic defendability was introduced by
   a) Davies b) Houston
   c) Brown d) Slater
66. Males having largest territories are called
   a) Polygynous b) Polyandrous
   c) Polygonus d) Polyandry
67. Smallest territories having males are called
   a) Polygynous b) Monogamous
   c) Bachelor d) Both b and c
68. Type of male's territory
   a) Leen system b) Let system
   c) Lean system d) Lek system
69. Territories also avoids
   a) Cannibalism b) Predatorism
   c) Commensalism d) Parasitism
70. Important result of territoriality is
   a) Population regression b) Population regulation
   c) Population suppression d) Population separation
71. Secondary functions of territorial behaviour
   a) Home range becomes familiar b) Able to escape from predators
   c) Reduces spread of diseases d) All
72. Superterritories mostly common in
   a) Polyandrous b) Polygamou
   c) Polygynou d) All
73. Social behaviour in animals are of
   a) Territorial rights
   b) Dominance and subordinate relationship
   c) Eadershi
   d) All
74. Which of the following sequence is most common in territorial hehaviour
   a) Threat,combat,advertisement b) Advertisement, threat, combat
   c) Combat,threat,advertisement d) Threat,advertisement, combat
75. Dominance hierarchies are most common when
   a) Resources are concentrated in one part of environment
   b) Males are larger than females
   c) There is no parental care
   d) Resources are uniformly distributed throughout the environment

76. The Norwegian biologists Thorleif Schjelderup-Ebbe made the first important observations on dominance on
    a) Cattle b) Hen
    c) Cat d) Dog
77. The strongest fish swims horizontally at about
    a) 20 degrees b) 32 degrees
    c) 2 degrees d) 45 degrees
78. Examples of the social dominance and dominance hierarchy
    a) Deer b) Elephant seals
    c) A only d) A & b
79. Type of hierarchy in rabbits
    a) Triangular hierarchy b) Simple linear hierarchy
    c) Two linear hierarchies d) None
80. Individuals have no memory of past encounters and fight every time they meet
    a) Statistical hierarchy b) Assessment hierarchy
    c) Confidence hierarchy d) All of the above
81. The act of winning a fight increases the vigour with which the victor enters its next encounter, so enhancing its chances of winning again and vice versa.
    a) Assessment hierarchy b) Confidence hierarchy
    c) Statistical hierarchy d) All of the above
82. Individuals use their memory of past encounters to decide which individuals they will fight and which they will avoid
    a) Confidence hierarchy b) Statistical hierarchy
    c) Assessment hierarchy d) A&b
83. Females are dominant to males in
    a) Hyenas b) Vervet monkeys
    c) None of the above d) A&b
84. Characteristics of territoriality
    a) Symmetric interspecific b) Asymmetric intraspecific
    c) Symmetric intraspecific d) Asymmetric interspecific
85. Which shape of territories would be of great advantage to territory owners
    a) Circular b) Triangular
    c) Square d) Hexagon
86. Female American bullfrogs (Rana *catesbeian*a) choose territories based on
    a) Territory size b) Type of vegetation
    c) Defended by older and large males d) All the above
87. Lek system of territory is observed in
    a) White-bearded mankin b) Hammer head bat
    c) Prairie chicken d) All the above

88. Unidirectional dominance relationship was seen in
    a) Cattle   b) Duroc
    c) A only   d) None of above
89. The sex difference was larger in
    a) Hampshire   b) Duroc
    c) Both   d) None of above
90. Dominance based not on individual recognition, but on badges of status that can be instantly recognized even by unfamiliar individuals is called
    a) Superior dominance   b) Badges of status
    c) A&b   d) None of the above
91. Badges of status observed in
    a) Rat   b) Hen
    c) Sparrows   d) Elephant
92. Whenever the behaviour of one animal is inhibited in the presence of another is called
    a) Dominance   b) Inferior
    c) Superior   d) None of the above
93. Ranking of dominant males in a single sequence, the system is called
    a) Assessment hierarchy
    b) Interspecific hierarchies
    c) Intraspecific hierarchies
    d) Simple and linear dominance hierarchy
94. Intraspecific and interspecific hierarchies are seen in
    a) Dunlins   b) Sparrow
    c) Titmice   d) Elephant
95. Type of hierarchy in Laboratory mice
    a) Intraspecific hierarchies   b) Confidence
    c) Assessment   d) Interspecific hierarchies
96. Type of hierarchy in sea anemone
    a) Confidence   b) Assessment
    c) Statistical hierarchy   d) All The Above
97. Assessment hierarchy is seen in
    a) Insects   b) Amphibians
    c) All The Above   d None of the above
98. Pseudo penile display is more common in
    a) Laboratory mice   b) Oyster-catchers
    c) Spotted hyenas   d Red-winged blackbirds
99. Good example of elastic disc territories
    a) North America dunlins   b) Sea anemone
    c) Spotted hyenas   d All the above

100. Males who are tolerated by territory owners in their territory for long periods to defend territory are called
   a) Dominant males
   b) Satellite males
   c) Submissive male
   d) None of the above
101. Example to study variations in economic value of territories
   a) Spotted hyenas
   b) Orange-rumped honey bees
   c) Sea anemone
   d) Oyster-catchers
102. Red-winged blackbirds attract to the males based on
   a) Body conformation
   b) Territory size
   c) Type of vegetation
   d) All the above
103. In orange-rumped honey bees, one male can copulate ______ different females.
   a) 30
   b) 18
   c) 20
   d) 15
104. In Lek system of territoriality females make comparison between male based on
   a) Posture of males
   b) Behaviour of males
   c) Display or sound that they make
   d) All the above
105. Secondary function of territoriality
   a) Reduction in the spread of parasites
   b) Reduction in the spread of
   c) All the aboove
   d) None of the above
106. Type of dominance relationship in swine
   a) Bidirectional
   b) Unidirectional
   c) Triangular
   d) All the above
107. Degree of reliability that they appear at first sight in badges of status
   a) Higher
   b) Lower
   c) Same
   d) None
108. The hierarchy in which no rank relationship exist between subordinates
   a) Statistical hierarchy
   b) Confidence
   c) Dominance hierarchy
   d) Assessment
109. Among the group of animals, the animal with least parasitic infestation usually become
   a) Submissive
   b) Dominant
   c) No importance
   d) Inferior
110. Dominance hierarchy of hens is arranged by
   a) Sex
   b) Age
   c) All the above
   d) None of the above
111. Territories can change in size and shape with
   a) Seasons
   b) Population
   c) Animals age
   d) All the above

112. Function of the territory system
   a) To attract the female to mate
   b) To be to act as a display area
   c) For the males leap in the air
   d) All the above
113. Breeding success in males depends on
   a) Territory size
   b) Type of vegetation in territory
   c) All the above
   d) None of the above
114. Mortality is less in territories which are defended by
   a) Small and juvenile males
   b) Large and older males
   c) Large and older fem
115. American jacana polyandrous female birds are ___________ per cent bigger than males.
   a) 70-80
   b) 50-70
   c) 20 -30
   d) 40-50
116. Small and no food is observed in the territories of
   a) Gulls
   b) Gannets
   c) Terns
   d) All the above
117. Relationship between barrows and gilts
   a) Barrows are more submissive than gilts
   b) Barrows are more dominant than gilts
   c) Equal positions
   d) No relationship
118. Relationship between Blue titmice and black-capped chickadees
   a) Blue titmice superior to the black-capped chickadees
   b) Blue titmice inferior to the black-capped chickadees
   c) Both are equal
   d) No relationship
119. The personality trait where in animal strives to attain and maintain status is called
   a) Competition
   b) Dominance
   c) Aggression
   d) Territoriality
120. Peck order in chicken is an example for
   a) Social structure
   b) Submissive behaviour
   c) Dominance hierarchies
   d) Territorial behaviour

Answer Key

1	c	2	c	3	a	4	a	5	c	6	d	7	a
8	a	9	c	10	b	11	a	12	c	13	b	14	c
15	a	16	a	17	d	18	d	19	b	20	d	21	d
22	a	23	a	24	b	25	c	26	a	27	c	28	b
29	d	30	a	31	a	32	c	33	b	34	d	35	a
36	c	37	a	38	b	39	d	40	a	41	a	42	b
43	d	44	c	45	b	46	c	47	d	48	c	49	b
50	d	51	c	52	a	53	b	54	c	55	d	56	a
57	c	58	d	59	d	60	b	61	c	62	a	63	c
64	b	65	c	66	a	67	c	68	d	69	a	70	b
71	d	72	a	73	d	74	b	75	a	76	b	77	c
78	d	79	c	80	a	81	b	82	c	83	d	84	b
85	d	86	c	87	d	88		89	a	90	b	91	c
92	a	93	d	94	c	95	b	96	c	97	c	98	c
99		100	b	101	d	102	d	103	b	104	c	105	c
106	a	107	a	108	c	109	b	110	c	111	d	112	d
113	c	114	b	115	b	116	d	117	b	118	a	119	b
120	c												

13

Homeostasis and Time Management

Soumosish Paul

Department of Zoology, Achaury Prafulla Chandra College, New Barrackpore Kolkata West Bengal.

Introduction

Homeostasis is unlike any time control process because it involves a very complicated relationship between fundamental knowledge of balance and coordination that ensures existence and performance of all creatures. It is in fact one of the major functioning mechanisms of biological systems, which allows them to sustain stable internal surroundings regardless of outside changes. This regulatory system is essential for evolutionary survival as well as physiological balance. At the same time, time management-often viewed in terms of human productivity-plays an important part in biology by influencing biological clocks and circadian rhythms. In order to be healthy, behavior and species evolution, physiological processes have to synchronize their daily and seasonal changes caused by environment factors. At first glance, these two concepts seem to be unrelated; but if viewed from the perspectives of biology and evolution, it becomes clear that they are deeply connected. These include temperature levels, pH values, and glucose concentrations among others that need to be maintained if life has to exist: homeostasis is necessary in order to keep these conditions stable. On the other hand, biological systems rely on time management especially through circadian rhythms so as to schedule diverse activities like feeding, sleeping metabolism or reproduction.This introduction describes how an organism manages to control and regulate its internal processes in conjunction with environmental stimuli is what makes it possible for organisms to live long, and perform productive activities and also enjoy a healthy life.In the year of 1926, Walter Cannon coined the word "homeostasis" with reference to a process through which all organisms maintain stable internal environments regardless changes happening outside their bodies. The theory's cornerstone was Claude Bernard's proposition of 'milieu intérieur', meaning moderate conditions needed for the existence of an organism itself the basic concept of homeostasis in physiology consists of the complex regulatory mechanisms regulating temperature, glucose metabolism, water balance, pH levels and other systems. Restoring equilibrium is achieved through perturbations that trigger some reactions from a reference point and mostly these are negative feedback loops for homeostatic processes. For instance, when pancreatic cells secrete insulin into the bloodstream after a meal because there is an increase in blood sugar level, insulin causes cells to absorb sugar thus restoring normal ranges.

Homeostasis plays a primary role in adaptation and survival, thus influencing the evolutionary direction of an organism. By enhancing an organism's ability to maintain homeostasis, the likelihood of its survival increases in the face of changing environmental conditions, resource acquisition and reproduction. Efficient homeostatic mechanisms assist animals to better cope with different types of stressors including temperature fluctuations, food shortages as well as diseases. Therefore, it is clear that homeostasis is not merely a means of maintaining stability; instead, it comprises dynamic actions that include monitoring, regulation and constant responses.

For managing health biological time, circadian rhythms are essential for keeping body normal functions in sync with outside world. By revolving round about once every twenty-four hours, these internal clocks known as circadian rhythms allow an organism to synchronize its physiological processes with day-night cycle. The master circadian clock located in suprachiasmatic nucleus (SCN) within hypothalamus modifies our body's rhythms depending information received from light sensitive retinal cells. Numerous biological processes such as hormone release, sleep-wake cycles, food habits and body temperature are regulated by this timer Within the context of biological organizations, time administration includes longer cycles like seasonal and ultradian rhythms (which occur multiple times in a day) along with daily circadian rhythm. It is important for existence since such activities have to correspond with such time forms. For instance, a good number of creatures go along with their breeding periods with seasonal alternations so that their young ones are produced when there are enough supplies. Similarly, respiration and heart rate are regulated through ultradian cycles for ensuring sustainable key body systems.

The ability of organisms to adjust to changes in their environment is ensured by the entrainment of circadian rhythms with external environmental cues. The entrainment of circadian rhythms is primarily stimulated by light; however, they can also be influenced by temperature, food availability and social interactions. It is this temporal alignment that makes homeostasis possible because it allows for synchronization of immunological, endocrine and metabolic processes with external environment. Circadian rhythm disturbance such as shift work, jet lag, irregular sleep patterns among others leads to homeostatic imbalance which increases susceptibility towards conditions like obesity, diabetes mellitus and cardiovascular diseases as well as mental disorders.

This synergy of time management with homeostasis is of high significance from an evolutionary perspective. Through history, organisms have evolved intricate systems for balancing internal environments and enhancing maximum interaction with external worlds. For instance, major alterations in the respiratory and thermoregulatory systems were necessary to facilitate the move from water to land so that demand for more variable conditions could be met. The life-threatening homeostasis processes on which these transformations are founded ensure self-preservation during the environmental revolutions.

Similarly, evolutionary improvements of circadian timers have enhanced chances for survival for living beings as they enable them to predict and react to regular changes in their surroundings such as switching between day time and night time or transitioning from summer to winter.

The importance of time management in relation to homeostasis emphasizes why our lives should be filled with lifestyle choices that promote excellent health and well-being. It is critical that these include eating healthy foods, getting enough sleep at night, being outside in daylight and engaging in regular physical activities. Notably, physical activity has profound effects on circadian rhythms and immune or metabolic functions resulting in improved balance of bodily systems. When people employ time management techniques that are in tandem with their biological clock, they work more efficiently, enhance self-esteem and minimize chances of contracting diseases In general, research into time management as well as homeostasis reveals a fundamental relationship that impacts human health, biology and evolution. Though they differ significantly, these actions are intimately linked to life and living systems. As such, new possibilities have emerged from the research which has opened up opportunities for better productivity, life understanding and health outcomes based on the complexes that control such activities. Time management and homeostatic regulation is a topic of extensive study with far-reaching consequences for various fields including biology and medicine among others.

MCQ's

1. What is homeostasis?
   a) The ability to maintain internal equilibrium.
   b) The ability to manage external changes.
   c) The ability to control social interactions.
   d) The process of energy conservation.
2. The term "homeostasis" was first used by whom?
   a) Claude Bernard b) Walter Cannon
   c) Robert Hooke d) Charles Darwin
3. Among the following, which is NOT a physiological component of homeostasis?
   a) Temperature b) Glucose levels
   c) Social interactions d) Water balance
4. Identify the option that most accurately describes how the hypothalamus controls circadian rhythms and homeostasis?
   a) It regulates emotional responses by releasing melatonin in response to social stress.
   b) It monitors light exposure and adjusts the circadian clock through the release of hormones like melatonin.
   c) It manages the body's glucose levels by directly influencing the respiratory and cardiovascular systems.
   d) It stimulates the production of digestive enzymes in response to changes in light and temperature.
5. Which hormone directly affects how long a person sleeps and wakes up?
   a) Cortisol b) Insulin
   c) Melatonin d) Adrenaline
6. How do circadian rhythms affect body temperature?
   a) They cause body temperature to rise at night and fall during the day.
   b) They maintain constant body temperature regardless of the time of day.
   c) Body temperature peaks in the late afternoon and declines at night.
   d) They fluctuate depending on physical activity, not the time of day.

7. Which natural cycles can an organism adapt to with the help of time management?
   a) Sleep cycles
   b) Light and dark cycles
   c) Hormone cycles
   d) Seasonal cycles
8. What is the main factor that influences circadian rhythms?
   a) Light exposure
   b) Eating patterns
   c) Exercise frequency
   d) Social behavior
9. What are the principal differences between thermoregulation and glucose regulation in the homeostasis feedback loop mechanism?
   a) Both rely on negative feedback, but thermoregulation involves hormonal responses, while glucose regulation involves muscular adjustments.
   b) Thermoregulation involves hormonal and behavioral responses, while glucose regulation involves the release of insulin and glucagon.
   c) Thermoregulation uses positive feedback to stabilize temperature, while glucose regulation relies on changes in blood pressure.
   d) Thermoregulation is governed by the cardiovascular system, whereas glucose regulation is controlled by neural feedback
10. What is the term for the synchronisation of circadian rhythms with external cues?
    a) Photic entrainment
    b) Thermoregulation
    c) Ultradian cycles
    d) Feedback inhibition
11. Among the following which involves for regulation of homeostasis?
    a) Internal stability
    b) External stimuli
    c) Time management
    d) Daily behavior patterns
12. Name the biological system that directly controls circadian rhythms?
    a) Digestive system
    b) Endocrine system
    c) Circulatory system
    d) Suprachiasmatic nucleus (SCN)
13. How often do cycles that are referred to as diurnal rhythms occur?
    a) Once per 24 hours
    b) Twice per day
    c) Every 6 hours
    d) Once per year
14. What is the main role of the suprachiasmatic nucleus (SCN) in relation to circadian rhythms and time regulation?
    a) It regulates cardiovascular responses during periods of increased physical activity.
    b) It adjusts the sleep-wake cycle by regulating the production of glucose in response to blood sugar levels.
    c) It coordinates the body's internal clock with external cues, such as light and darkness, influencing physiological cycles.
    d) It controls the production of insulin and glucagon based on environmental light patterns.

15. What possible effects can result from disrupting the synchronization of circadian cycles, and how is light exposure during the day affected by this?
    a) Light exposure suppresses melatonin production, helping maintain wakefulness; disruption can lead to metabolic imbalances and mood disorders.
    b) Light exposure enhances the release of cortisol, which synchronizes the sleep-wake cycle; disruption can lead to increased cardiovascular activity.
    c) Light exposure regulates glucose metabolism, preventing energy imbalances; disruption leads to hyperactivity and reduced sleep.
    d) Light exposure triggers adrenaline release, preparing the body for physical activity; disruption can lead to glucose regulation disorders.
16. What kind of the role of the suprachiasmatic nucleus (SCN)?
    a) Controlling reproductive cycles
    b) Regulating body temperature during exercise
    c) Synchronizing circadian rhythms with light-dark cycles
    d) Stimulating glucose production
17. Which kind of process is primarily regulated by infradian rhythms?
    a) Daily sleep-wake cycles
    b) Monthly reproductive cycles
    c) Rapid digestion of food
    d) Moment-to-moment changes in heart rate
18. What role does the immune system play in homeostasis?
    a) Regulating glucose levels
    b) Eliminating infections
    c) Controlling hormone levels
    d) Maintaining body temperature
19. "Ultradian rhythm" refers to?
    a) Rhythms longer than 24 hours
    b) Rhythms shorter than 24 hours
    c) Seasonal rhythms
    d) Rhythms related to circadian cycles
20. The relationship between the endocrine system and homeostatic regulation can be best described by which of the following?
    a) The endocrine system primarily stabilizes internal temperature through the release of neurotransmitters from the hypothalamus.
    b) The endocrine system manages energy homeostasis by regulating metabolic hormones such as insulin, glucagon, and cortisol.
    c) The endocrine system is responsible for maintaining water balance by increasing blood pressure in response to hormonal cues.
    d) The endocrine system directly controls heart rate during circadian disruptions through the release of adrenaline.

21. Which statement correctly compares ultradian and infradian rhythms in relation to circadian rhythms?
   a) Ultradian rhythms occur less frequently than circadian rhythms, while infradian rhythms occur more frequently.
   b) Both ultradian and infradian rhythms are governed by the suprachiasmatic nucleus (SCN) and rely on external cues like temperature and light.
   c) Ultradian rhythms occur more frequently than circadian rhythms, whereas infradian rhythms occur less frequently, often involving reproductive or seasonal cycles.
   d) Ultradian rhythms are primarily responsible for regulating sleep patterns, while infradian rhythms control stress responses

22. How does melatonin affect the sleep-wake cycle?
   a) It increases alertness during the day.
   b) It signals the body to initiate sleep at night.
   c) It stimulates energy production at night.
   d) It reduces the need for sleep during the night

23. What role do ultradian rhythms play in biological regulation?
   a) They regulate processes that occur less frequently than once per day.
   b) They regulate processes that occur more frequently than once per day.
   c) They control seasonal reproductive cycles.
   d) They synchronize circadian rhythms with the environment.

24. How do seasonal variations in light exposure influence the body's homeostatic mechanisms and circadian rhythms?
   a) Increased light exposure during winter months leads to reduced melatonin production, improving sleep and mood.
   b) Reduced light exposure in winter months disrupts circadian rhythms, affecting hormone release and energy balance.
   c) Seasonal variations in light exposure enhance thermoregulation, allowing better adaptation to colder temperatures.
   d) Seasonal changes in light exposure have minimal impact on homeostasis and circadian regulation, as these processes remain constant

25. Which of the following disrupts circadian rhythms?
   a) Poor time management
   b) Increased light exposure
   c) Adequate sleep
   d) Efficient exercise routines

26. The main biological clock of the body is located in which brain region?
   a) Cerebellum
   b) Amygdala
   c) Suprachiasmatic nucleus (SCN)
   d) Hippocampus

27. What is the primary role of the hypothalamus in homeostasis?
   a) Stimulating hunger
   b) Regulating body temperature
   c) Controlling emotional responses
   d) Influencing speech patterns

28. What role does the interaction between circadian rhythms and mood regulation play in seasonal affective disorder (SAD)?
    a) SAD is caused by increased melatonin production during winter months, leading to heightened activity levels.
    b) SAD occurs when reduced light exposure disrupts circadian rhythms, causing imbalances in melatonin and serotonin production.
    c) SAD is triggered by excessive sunlight during summer months, leading to an overproduction of stress hormones.
    d) SAD is a result of circadian rhythm enhancement during colder months, leading to improved emotional stability
29. What is the effect of light exposure on melatonin production, and how does this interaction impact sleep-wake cycles?
    a) Light exposure decreases melatonin production, leading to increased alertness during the day and sleep initiation at night.
    b) Light exposure enhances melatonin production, promoting sleep during daylight hours and wakefulness at night.
    c) Light exposure has no direct effect on melatonin production, which remains constant regardless of environmental changes.
    d) Light exposure disrupts melatonin production, causing irregular sleep-wake cycles and mood disorders
30. Which of the following describes how infradian rhythms differ from circadian rhythms in terms of biological regulation?
    a) Infradian rhythms regulate body temperature, while circadian rhythms control glucose metabolism.
    b) Infradian rhythms occur on a monthly or seasonal basis, influencing processes like reproduction, while circadian rhythms occur daily.
    c) Infradian rhythms are primarily responsible for regulating sleep cycles, while circadian rhythms manage daily emotional responses.
    d) Infradian rhythms affect short-term changes in blood pressure, whereas circadian rhythms regulate long-term metabolic cycles.
31. Which of the following best describes circadian rhythm disruption?
    a) It causes increased body temperature throughout the day.
    b) It can lead to sleep disorders and metabolic imbalances.
    c) It improves glucose regulation.
    d) It reduces stress responses.
32. Which biological cycle lasts more than 24 hours?
    a) Circadian rhythm b) Ultradian rhythm
    c) Infradian rhythm d) Diurnal rhythm
33. What kind of rhythm governs sleep and wakefulness cycles in humans?
    a) Ultradian rhythm b) Diurnal rhythm
    c) Circadian rhythm d) Infradian rhythm

34. What happens if irregular light exposure throws off circadian rhythms?
    a) Glucose regulation improves.
    b) Sleep patterns may become irregular.
    c) Hormonal production is stabilized.
    d) Melatonin production increases.
35. Which of the following influences the synchronization of circadian rhythms?
    a) Diet
    b) Social media
    c) Physical exercise
    d) Both a and c
36. How do circadian rhythms affect the body's thermoregulatory response during the day and night?
    a) Body temperature is maintained at constant levels throughout the day, but decreases sharply at night to conserve energy.
    b) Thermoregulation follows a circadian rhythm, with body temperature peaking in the late afternoon and declining during the night.
    c) The body's thermoregulatory response is entirely dependent on external temperature changes and remains unaffected by circadian rhythms.
    d) Body temperature increases at night to aid digestion, while circadian rhythms suppress this response during the day
37. Which of the following best explains the consequence of circadian rhythm disruption on the body's homeostatic balance?
    a) Disrupted circadian rhythms cause elevated insulin levels, leading to improved glucose regulation.
    b) Disrupted circadian rhythms lead to hormonal imbalances, metabolic disorders, and increased risk of mood-related diseases.
    c) Disrupted circadian rhythms enhance thermoregulation, allowing better adaptation to extreme temperatures.
    d) Disrupted circadian rhythms improve the synchronization of metabolic and digestive functions with physical activity
38. How do circadian rhythms affect the body's thermoregulatory response during the day and night?
    a) Body temperature is maintained at constant levels throughout the day, but decreases sharply at night to conserve energy.
    b) Thermoregulation follows a circadian rhythm, with body temperature peaking in the late afternoon and declining during the night.
    c) The body's thermoregulatory response is entirely dependent on external temperature changes and remains unaffected by circadian rhythms.
    d) Body temperature increases at night to aid digestion, while circadian rhythms suppress this response during the day
39. What is one consequence of inefficient time management in biological systems?
    a) Improved health
    b) Disruption of homeostasis
    c) Increase in productivity
    d) Enhanced metabolic rate

40. The circadian system is particularly sensitive to which environmental factor?
   a) Sound
   b) Redox state
   c) Touch
   d) Humidity levels

41. Exercise can help reset what type of rhythm?
   a) Diurnal rhythm
   b) Circadian rhythm
   c) Ultradian rhythm
   d) Infradian rhythm

42. What is the relationship between homeostasis and circadian rhythms in regulating body temperature and metabolic rate during different times of the day?
   a) Homeostasis ensures constant body temperature throughout the day, while circadian rhythms adjust metabolic rates according to glucose levels.
   b) Homeostasis adjusts both body temperature and metabolic rate according to external light exposure, while circadian rhythms remain stable.
   c) Circadian rhythms influence body temperature and metabolic rate, with body temperature dropping at night, while homeostasis maintains this balance.
   d) Circadian rhythms control body temperature in response to eating patterns, while homeostasis maintains glucose levels through negative feedback

43. What can disrupt the body's homeostatic balance?
   a) Constant adaptation
   b) Immune system disorders
   c) Low oxygen concentration
   d) Efficient time management

44. A rhythm that takes place less than once a day is referred to as what?
   a) Circadian rhythm
   b) Diurnal rhythm
   c) Infradian rhythm
   d) Ultradian rhythm

45. How does seasonal changes of biological systems play a critical role in animal survival, particularly in seasonal environments?
   a) It enables animals to synchronize reproductive cycles and energy conservation with the availability of food resources.
   b) It allows animals to regulate blood pressure and heart rate based on changing temperatures and seasonal shifts.
   c) It enhances neural adaptation to seasonal changes, promoting increased social behaviors during summer months.
   d) It ensures stable glucose levels by regulating feeding behaviors across varying seasons

46. In what way does the body's circadian clock influence cardiovascular function, particularly in response to external environmental cues?
   a) The circadian clock reduces cardiovascular activity during daylight hours to conserve energy for nighttime activities.
   b) The circadian clock increases heart rate in response to light exposure, optimizing blood flow and oxygen delivery during waking hours.
   c) The circadian clock prevents fluctuations in blood pressure by maintaining constant cardiovascular output throughout the day.
   d) The circadian clock regulates hormone release, influencing heart rate and blood pressure according to physical activity levels.

47. Time management plays an important role in maintaining what biological process?
    a) Blood glucose levels
    b) Circadian rhythm synchronization
    c) Hair growth
    d) Skin hydration
48. Seasonal cycles are associated with which biological rhythm?
    a) Ultradian rhythm
    b) Infradian rhythm
    c) Diurnal rhythm
    d) Circadian rhythm
49. What is a significant outcome of effective time management in biological systems?
    a) Increased stress
    b) Synchronization with circadian rhythms
    c) Disruption of homeostasis
    d) Increase in blood pressure
50. The SCN uses what mechanism to regulate circadian rhythm?
    a) Neural connections
    b) Diffusion of light
    c) Sound waves
    d) Water regulation.

Answer Key

1	a	2	b	3	c	4	b	5	c	6	c	7	b
8	a	9	b	10	a	11	a	12	d	13	a	14	c
15	a	16	c	17	b	18	b	19	b	20	b	21	c
22	b	23	b	24	b	25	b	26	c	27	b	28	b
29	a	30	b	31	b	32	c	33	c	34	b	35	d
36	b	37	b	38	b	39	b	40	b	41	b	42	c
43	b	44	d	45	a	46	b	47	b	48	b	49	b
50	a												

14

Circadian Clock

***Pramod Kumar*[1] *and Rajesh Kumar*[2]**

[1]*Department of Veterinary Physiology & Biochemisry*

[2]*Department of Veterinary Gynaecology and Obstetrics*

College of Veterinary Science & Animal Husbandry, Acharya Narendra Deva University of Agriculture & Technology, Ayodhya, Uttar Pradesh

Introduction

The development of the domestic phenotype mirrors the domestication process. Are certain behavioral patterns typically lost when animal are domesticated? Why do domesticated animals exhibit some behaviors more frequently than their wild counterparts? Darwin (1868) believed that in captivity biological traits are lost through disuse. Hemmer (1990) proposed that domestic animals have experienced a kind of regressive evolution, in which their behavior is less influence by environmental stimuli than that of their wild counterparts. The Earth's rotation around its axis influences our physiology and behaviour. Animal species that are compelled to be active continuously typically exhibit poor performance, health, and survival. However, we examine the evidence of animals displaying extended periods of activity with weakened or nonexistent circadian rhythms and no observable negative consequences. Available reports suggested that there is a greater prevalence of around-the-clock and ultradian activity patterns than commonly acknowledged.

This is especially true among herbivores, animals in Polar Regions and constant physical environments, animals in specific life-history stages, and highly social animals. Various mechanisms exist, but research indicates that certain circadian pacemakers still function in animals that are active throughout the day and night. The prevalence of continuous activity in various animals and habitats, along with a wide range of underlying mechanisms, suggests a pattern of convergent evolution. The circadian system's organizational principles and complexity allow for potential chrono-biological plasticity. There could be compromises between the advantages of consistent daily patterns and adaptability, which, due to reasons that are not well comprehended, result in the functional suitability of irregular daily patterns only in specific environments and for specific ways of life.

The study of animal behaviour in their natural habitat is known as Ethology. Behaviour is a co-ordination between nervous system and locomotion i.e. the response of an animal to the external stimuli that can be seen and analysed by the other individual animal. It can also be defined as an expressed sum of individual muscle contractions and hormonal secretions. The limbic system is that part of brain which is involved in behavioural and emotional responses.

The structures of limbic system buried deep within the brain, underneath the cerebral cortex and above the brainstem. The thalamus, hypothalamus and basal ganglia are involved in the actions of the limbic system, but two of the major structures are the hippocampus and the amygdala Behaviour alters an animals' relationship to its external world, one of the principal consequences of behaviour is adjustment of the sensory input.

MCQ's

1. Study of behavior is known as_________
   a) Biology b) Ethology
   c) Psychlogy d) Ecology
2. The body circadium rhythm is regulated by
   a) Thymus b) Thyriod
   c) Pineal d) Pituitary
3. A woman"s menstrual cycle is an example of
   a) Cicadiam rhythm b) Infradian rhythm
   c) Ultradian rhythm d) All of the above
4. Courtship behavior of animal come in
   a) Imprinting b) Innate
   c) Classical conditioning d) None of the above
5. The period (cycle length) of circadian rhythms is determined
   a) Mostly by physical interaction between FRQ and CK1a
   b) Mostly by nature (history of environmental expoxure)
   c) Equally by and nature and nurture
   d) All the above
6. Coprophagy behaviour is found in___________
   a) Dog b) Cow
   c) Rabbit d) Goat
7. Wallowing behavior is found in__________
   a) Cow b) Buffalo
   c) Sheep d) All of the above
8. An example of associative learning would be
   a) Classical conditioning b) Operant conditioning
   c) Pavlovian conditioning d) All of the above
9. A songbird that hears the songs of other species as well as its own
   a) Will sing the song of other species, but needs prefer own song
   b) Will instinctively sing the song of its species perfectly
   c) Will sing other songs as well as its own
   d) Will be confused and not master any song

10. The level of specificity of signals may be
    a) Species-specific
    b) Individual specific
    c) Anonymous
    d) All of the above
11. Increased response to an increase in light intensity is called
    a) Positive phototaxic
    b) Kinesis
    c) Negative phototaxic
    d) Luminis
12. Which of the following is an example of a question about the ultimate causation of a behavior?
    a) What muscles are involved when a humming bird hovers over a flower?
    b) When is the critical period for imprinting in young goats?
    c) Which hormones must be present at what levels to make a female lizard receptive to male courtship?
    d) None of the above
13. Which of the following involves trial-and-error learning?
    a) Habituation
    b) Classical conditioning
    c) Sensitization
    d) Operant conditioning
14. Human behavior, like other mammalian behavior, is determined
    a) Strictly by the genes
    b) Strictly by learning
    c) By a mixture of genes and learning
    d) None of the above
15. Learning to not respond to a stimulus is called
    a) Imprinting
    b) Sensitization
    c) Kinesis
    d) Habituation
16. A goose retrieving a stray egg and rolling it back into its nest is an example of
    a) Instinctive behavior
    b) Operaant conditioning
    c) Associative behavior
    d) Learning preparedness
17. A "Skinner box" is used for experiments in
    a) Classical conditioning
    b) Operant conditioning
    c) Migration
    d) Taxis
18. A rat that is "maze-dull"
    a) Will pass on that trait to its offspring
    b) Can never learn anything else either
    c) Both of the above
    d) None of the above
19. Chemical signals between individuals of the same species are called
    a) Endogenous
    b) Hormones
    c) Kinesis
    d) Pheromone
20. The component of an animal's nervous system that provides the instruction for carrying out a particular fixed action pattern is called a(n)
    a) Sign stimulus
    b) Stimulus/response chain
    c) Innate releasing mechanism
    d) Exogenous biological clock

21. All the thousands of human languages are based on the same set of how many consonant sounds?
    a) 26 b) 40
    c) 4 d) 260
22. How many of the basic consonant sounds can a normal human baby distinguish?
    a) Half of them
    b) One
    c) It depends on the child's ethnic background
    d) All of them
23. A sensitive phase and critical period are associated with what type of behavior?
    a) Cognitive b) Kinesis
    c) Imprinting d) Taxis
24. Which of the following animals is a brood parasite?
    a) Anolis lizards b) Love birds
    c) Fruit flies d) Cuckoos
25. Circadian rhythms are based on approximately a
    a) 24-hours b) 2-hours
    c) 30 days d) 7 days
26. The biological clock of mammals is located in the
    a) Suprachiasmatic nuclei of the pineal gland
    b) Suprachiasmatic nuclei of the hypothalamus
    c) Androgens of gonads
    d) Melatonin of pineal gland
27. Nonoriented changes in activity level or movement are called
    a) Exogenous b) Kinesis
    c) Taxis d) Migration
    e) Conspecific
28. How is the distance to a food source communicated by a dancing honeybee?
    a) By how far it moves during the straight run portion of the dance
    b) By the direction it waggles its abdomen
    c) By which direction it turns after making the straight run
    d) By the tempo or degree of vigor of the dance
29. Dog salivating at the sound of a can opener.
    a) Fixed conditioning b) Classical conditioning
    c) Habituation d) Imprinting
    e) Operant conditioning
30. Humans ignoring night sounds while a sleep.
    a) Classical conditioning b) Fixed-action pattern
    c) Operant conditioning d) Habituation

31. A rat in a box learns to associate pressing a lever with obtaining food.
    a) Fixed conditioning
    b) Classical conditioning
    c) Imprinting
    d) Operant conditioning
32. Chemical messengers that are used for communication within an animal species are called
    a) Hormones
    b) Genes
    c) Pheromone
    d) Enzyme
33. Courtship behaviors in animals involve all of the following except:
    a) Visual cues
    b) Chemical signals
    c) Auditory cues
    d) All of the above involve courtship behavior
34. Circadian rhythm is controlled by a group of cells in the
    a) Central nervous system
    b) Brain stem
    c) Pituitary gland
    d) Hypothalamus
35. Hormone that is secreted to help in with sleep is called
    a) Dopamine
    b) Melatonin
    c) Serotonin
    d) Progestrone
36. Circadian rhythm a cycle based on a _________time period
    a) 12 hours
    b) 16 hours
    c) 24 hours
    d) 12 and 24 hours
37. How long ago was reliable evidence for the existence of endogenous (internal) 24-hour rhythmicity first recorded in an animal?
    a) 10 years
    b) 25 years
    c) 50 years
    d) 100 years
38. The word "circadian" was not created until the 1950's. Who introduced the word?
    a) Colin Pittendrigh
    b) Franz Halberg
    c) Jürgen Aschoff
    d) Albert Einstein
39. Study the ecological effect of animal behavior called
    a) Behavior ecology
    b) Comparative psychology
    c) Ethology
    d) Socio-biology
40. Evolution of social behavior in animal is called
    a) Ethology
    b) Comparative psychology
    c) Socio-biology
    d) Anthropomorphism
41. The period (cycle length) of circadian rhythms is determined by
    a) Mostly by nature (genetic inheritance)
    b) Mostly by nurture (history of environmental exposure)
    c) Equally by nature and nurture
    d) By neither nature nor nurture

42. According to the "non-parametric theory of entrainment", entrainment (synchronization) of circadian rhythms by environmental stimuli is achieved by
    a) The slowing down or speeding up of the clock
    b) Discrete daily phase shifts
    c) Little green men hiding behind the bushes
    d) Genetic maturation
43. What is "food-anticipatory activity"?
    a) The preprandial secretion of insulin
    b) The postprandial secretion of saliva
    c) The expression of displeasure about a meal
    d) A psychological phenomenon related to expectation of outcomes
44. How long ago is circadian rhythmicity believed to have evolved?
    a) Several trillion years
    b) Several billion years
    c) Several million years
    d) Several thousand years
    e) Several hundred years
45. Why are nocturnal organisms active at night?
    a) Because their eyes are specialized for night vision
    b) Because their circadian system is unresponsive to light
    c) Because their active phase is genetically timed to subjective night
    d) A and C option
46. Sleep is controlled by
    a) By a homeostatic (restorative) system
    b) By the circadian system
    c) By both a homeostatic system and the circadian system
    d) By neither a homeostatic system nor the circadian system
47. The circadian system of mammals is sensitive to ambient illumination that reaches
    a) The rods and cones in the retina of the eye
    b) Specialized photosensitive ganglion cells in the retina
    c) The skin
    d) Both a and b
48. The "master circadian pacemaker" in the mammalian brain is located in the
    a) Suprachiasmatic nucleus
    b) Preoptic area
    c) Thalamus
    d) Hippocampus
49. The suprachiasmatic nucleus can be anatomically and functionally subdivided into two regions. These two regions differ because
    a) One is mostly ventrally located whereas the other is mostly dorsally located
    b) One is the target of many projections from extra- hypothalamic sites whereas the other is not
    c) One contains many intrinsically-rhythmic neurons whereas the other contains few
    d) All of the above

50. The molecular mechanism responsible for circadian rhythmicity can best be characterized as
    a) Being part of the cell cycle
    b) Consisting of a single translational loop
    c) Being a feedbackless process
    d) Consisting of one or more transcriptional/translational loops
51. The change of behavior of life experience of is called
    a) Instinct b) Matauration
    c) Learning d) Imprinting
52. A persistent phase delay of the internal clock is most likely the cause of which of these diseases?
    a) Lung cancer b) Syphilis
    c) Sleep-onset insomnia d) Delayed sleep phase syndrome
53. In a adult cow, an rectal temperature of 38.0–39.3 ^{0}C(100.4–102.8 ^{0}F) Clearly indicates a state of fever
    a) Is suggestive of fever at night but not in the afternoon
    b) Provides no helpful information for the diagnosis of fever
    c) Clearly indicates the absence of fever
    d) None of the above
54. Circadian rhythm effect human which are following
    a) Sleep pattern b) Blood pressure
    c) Hormone release d) All of the above
55. What is the term "circadian rhythm" associated with
    a) Body clock b) Heart beat
    c) Movement of merry go round d) Movement of pendulum
56. Animals that are awake during the day are
    a) Nocturnal b) Circadian
    c) Jet-lagged d) Diurnal
57. Which is best describe the "circadian rhythm"
    a) A 12 hours biological cycle b) A 48 hours biological cycle
    c) A 24 hours biological cycle d) The rotation of earth around sun
58. Which is true about biological clock
    a) We know a lot of about them
    b) They adjust with changing temperature
    c) They are depend on endogenous and linked with external cues
    d) They are easily disrupted
59. What is definition of biological rhythm
    a) The sleep wake cycle
    b) An internal response to change in your environment

c) Distinct pattern changes in body activity that confirm to cyclical time period
d) When you play a drum on your friend' belly

60. The sleep wake cycle a example of
a) Circadian Rhythm
b) Exogenous Zeitgeber
c) Ultradian Rhythm
d) Infradian Rhythm

61. Which of the following behaviors can be easily observed?
a) Pheromone release
b) Vocalizations
c) Ovulation
d) Mating dance

62. What does it mean to hibernate?
a) To change your physical characteristics
b) To sleep for an extended period of time during the winter
c) To travel to a warmer location
d) To eat all the oreos

63. Some adaptation are used to____________animals from their enemies
a) Share
b) Protect
c) Help
d) None of the above

64. Which of the following list of animals and their shelter is WRONG
a) Lion-Den
b) Dog-Kennel
c) Cow-Shed
d) Horse-borrow

65. Which of the following animal is an omnivores
a) Lion
b) Tigor
c) Bear
d) Deer

66. Which of the following animal is swallow its food as whole
a) Lion
b) Snake
c) Bear
d) Horse

67. Animal that chew the cud are mostly
a) Carnivores
b) Omnivores
c) Herbivores
d) All of the above

68. A rat that is "maze-dull"
a) Will pass on that trait to its offspring
b) Can never learn anything else either
c) Both of the above
d) None of the above

69. A female cat in heat urinates more often and in many places. Male cats congregate near the urine deposits and fight with each other. Which of the following is a proximate cause of this behavior of increased urination?
a) It announces to the males that she is in heat
b) Female cat that did not this in the past attracted more males
c) It is result of hormonal changes associated with her reproductive cycle
d) The female cat learned the behavior from observing other

70. Which of the following is a behavioral pattern that results from a proximate cause?
   a) A cat kills a mouse to obtain food
   b) A male sheep fights with another male because it helps it to improve its social position and find a mate
   c) A goose squats and freezes motionless because that behavior helps it to escape a predator
   d) A female bird lays eggs because the amount of daylight is decreasing slightly each day
71. Which of the following is a behavioral pattern resulting from an ultimate cause?
   a) A male robin attacks a red tennis ball because it resemble the breast of another male
   b) A male robin attacks a red tennis ball because it confuses it with an encroaching male who will steal its territory
   c) A male robin attacks a red tennis ball because hormonal changes in spring increase its aggression
   d) A male robin attacks a red tennis ball because a part of its brain is stimulated by red objects
72. The proximate causes of behavior are interactions with the environment, but behavior is ultimately shaped by
   a) Hormones b) Evolution
   c) Sexuality d) Pheromone
73. Which of the following group of scientists is closely associated with ethology?
   a) Watson, Crick and Franklin b) McClintock, Goodall and Lyon
   c) Von Frisch, Lorenz and Chase d) Hardy, Weinberg and Castle
74. Animal communication involves what type of sensory information?
   a) Visual b) Auditory
   c) Chemical d) All of the above
75. What type of signal is long-lasting and works at night?
   a) Olfactory b) Visual
   c) Auditory d) Tactile
76. What type of signal is brief and can work at night or among obstructions?
   a) Olfactory b) Visual
   c) Auditory d) Tactile
77. What type of signal is fast and can requires daylight with no obstructions?
   a) Olfactory b) Visual
   c) Auditory d) Tactile
78. A chemical produced by an animal that serves as a communication to another animal of the same species is called
   a) A marker b) A inducer
   c) A pheromone d) A imprinter

79. Feeding behavior with a high energy intake-to-expenditure ratio is called
   a) Herbivory b) Autotrophy
   c) Hetrotrophy d) Optimal Foraging

80. Animals tend to maximize their energy intake-to-expenditure ratio. What is this behavior called?
   a) Optimal Foraging b) Agnostic behavior
   c) Dominance hierarchies d) Animal cognition

81. Which of the following is least related to the others?
   a) Ritual b) Agnostic behavior
   c) Dominance hierarchies d) Cognitive maps

82. Which of the following is least related to the others?
   a) Fixed-action pattern b) Classical conditioning
   c) Operant conditioning d) Habituation

83. Sparrows are receptive to learning songs only during a sensitive period. What term best applies to this behavior?
   a) Sign stimulus b) Imprinting
   c) Habituation d) Classical conditioning

84. A guinea pig loves the lettuce kept in the refrigerator and squeals each time the refrigerator door opens. What term best applies to this behavior?
   a) Sign stimulus b) Imprinting
   c) Habituation d) Classical conditioning

85. Parental protective behavior in turkeys is triggered by the cheeping sound of young chicks. What term best applies to this behavior?
   a) Sign stimulus b) Imprinting
   c) Habituation d) Classical conditioning

86. A salmon returns to its home stream to spawn. What term best applies to this behavior?
   a) Sign stimulus b) Imprinting
   c) Habituation d) Classical conditioning

87. Male insects attempt to mate with orchids but eventually stop responding to them. What term best applies to this behavior?
   a) Sign stimulus b) Imprinting
   c) Habituation d) Classical conditioning

88. Which of the following statements about learning and behavior is incorrect?
   a) Operant conditioning involves associating a behavior with a regard or punishment.
   b) Associative learning involves linking one stimulus with another.
   c) Classical conditioning involves trial-and-error learning.
   d) Behavior can be modified by learning, but some apparent learning is due to maturation.

89. Some dogs love attention, and Frodo the beagle learns that if he barks, he gets attention. Which of the following might you use to describe this behavior?
   a) Fixed-action pattern b) Classical conditioning
   c) Operant conditioning d) Social behavior
90. The type of learning that causes specially trained dogs to salivate when they hear bells is called
   a) Imprinting b) Classical conditioning
   c) Insight d) Habituation
91. Learning in which an associated stimulus may be used to elicit the same behavioral response as the original sign stimulus is called
   a) Classical conditioning b) Imprinting
   c) Operant conditioning d) Habituation
92. Loss of responsiveness to stimuli that convey little or no new information is called
   a) Classical b) Imprinting
   c) Adapting d) Habituation
93. You turn on a light and observe cockroaches scurrying to dark hiding places. What have you observed?
   a) Learned behavior b) Migration
   c) Taxis d) Visual communication
94. From which stage of sleep would it be thc easiest to wake someone up?
   a) Stage 1 b) Stage 2
   c) Stage 3 d) REM
95. Which stage of sleep is characterized by sleep spindle?
   a) Stage 1 b) Stage 2
   c) Stage 3 d) REM
96. What term do sleep researcher use designated stages 1-4 sleep?
   a) Deep sleep b) Paradoxical sleep
   c) Non-REM sleep d) REM sleep
97. Jet-lag is typically the worst when travelling
   a) North b) East
   c) West d) South
98. Freud called the hidden meaning of a dream__________content
   a) Surface b) Unconscious
   c) Latent d) Manifest
99. According to Freud, the visible or directly observable content of a dream is its----- content
   a) Primary b) Secondary
   c) Manifest d) Latent

100. A full sleep cycle (from stage 1 to REM) last approximately

a) 20 min. b) 6-8 hrs.

c) 90-100 min. d) 8-10 hrs.

Answer Key

1	b	2	c	3	b	4	b	5	a	6	c	7	b
8	c	9	a	10	d	11	a	12	d	13	d	14	c
15	d	16	a	17	b	18	a	19	d	20	c	21	b
22	d	23	c	24	d	25	a	26	b	27	b	28	b
29	b	30	d	31	d	32	c	33	d	34	d	35	b
36	c	37	d	38	b	39	c	40	c	41	a	42	b
43	a	44	b	45	d	46	c	47	d	48	a	49	d
50	d	51	c	52	d	53	c	54	d	55	a	56	d
57	c	58	c	59	c	60	a	61	b	62	b	63	b
64	d	65	c	66	b	67	c	68	a	69	c	70	d
71	b	72	b	73	c	74	d	75	a	76	c	77	b
78	c	79	d	80	a	81	d	82	a	83	b	84	d
85	a	86	b	87	c	88	c	89	c	90	b	91	a
92	d	93	c	94	a	95	b	96	c	97	b	98	c
99	c	100	c